Collins *gem*

GI

D0434659

This book has been compiled with the assistance of hundreds of brand-name manufacturers. Other sources are listed on page 59.

HarperCollins Publishers
Westerhill Road, Bishopbriggs, Glasgow G64 2QT

www.collins.co.uk

This edition published 2005

Reprint 10 9 8 7 6 5 4 3 2 1

© HarperCollins Publishers 2005

ISBN 0-00-721139-2

Editorial by Grapevine Publishing Services, London
Design by Judith Ash

Printed in Italy by Amadeus S.r.l.

CONTENTS

INTRODUCTION 8

BAKERY 62

Bread 63
Rolls 64
Tea Breads, Buns, Pastries 65
Cakes and Cream Cakes 66

BAKING PRODUCTS 68

Baking Agents 69
Fats 70
Mixes 70
Sundries 71

BEANS, PULSES AND CEREALS 72

Beans and Pulses 73
Cereals 75

BISCUITS, CRACKERS AND CRISPBREADS 76

Sweet Biscuits 77
Crackers and Crispbreads 78

BREAKFAST CEREALS AND CEREAL BARS 80

Breakfast Cereals 81

Hot Cereals 82

Muesli 83

Cereal Bars 84

CONDIMENTS, SAUCES AND GRAVY 86

Table Sauces 87

Mustards 88

Pickles and Chutneys 88

Salad Dressings 90

Vinegars 91

Cooking Sauces 91

Stock Cubes 92

Gravy Granules 93

DAIRY 94

Milk and Cream 95

Yoghurt and Fromage Frais 96

Butter and Margarine 98

Spreads 98

Cheeses 99

Cheese Spreads and Processed Cheese 102

DESSERTS AND PUDDINGS 104

Puddings 105

Sweet Pies and Flans   106
Chilled and Frozen Desserts   107
Toppings and Sauces   108

DRINKS   **110**

Alcoholic   111
Juices and Cordials   113
Fizzy Drinks   115
Hot and Milky Drinks   116

EGGS   **118**

FISH AND SEAFOOD   **120**

Fish and Seafood   121
Breaded, Battered or in Sauces   125

FRUIT   **126**

JAMS, MARMALADES AND SPREADS   **132**

Jams and Marmalades   133
Nut Butters   135
Savoury Spreads and Pastes   136

MEAT AND POULTRY   **138**

Cooked Meats   139
Cold Meats   143

OILS AND FATS — **146**

PASTA AND PIZZA — **148**

Pasta — 149
Pasta Sauces — 150
Canned Pasta — 150
Pasta Ready Meals — 151
Pizza — 152

PIES AND QUICHES — **154**

RICE AND NOODLES — **156**

SNACKS, NIBBLES AND DIPS — **158**

Crisps — 159
Nibbles — 160
Dried Fruit — 161
Nuts and Seeds — 162
Dips — 164

SOUP — **166**

Canned Soups — 167
Sachet/Cup Soups — 170

SUGAR AND SWEETENERS — **174**

SWEETS AND CHOCOLATES — **176**

VEGETABLES 184

VEGETARIAN 194

FAST FOOD 200

SOME GI COMPARISONS 208

MENU IDEAS FOR A LOW GI DIET 212

EATING OUT 217

British 218

Chinese 219

French 220

Greek 222

Indian 223

Italian 224

Japanese 226

Mexican 227

Middle Eastern 228

Spanish 230

Thai 231

Packed Lunches 232

FURTHER READING 236

USEFUL WEBSITES 238

USEFUL ADDRESSES 239

INTRODUCTION

For decades, dieters have been searching for the holy grail – a diet that helps them to lose weight and keep it off, that doesn't require constant weighing, measuring and counting, and doesn't leave them feeling too deprived. After all this time, could the GI diet finally provide the answer? Or is it just part of a much bigger picture?

Most diets work by limiting your intake of a particular food group – either carbohydrates, proteins or fat – while filling you up with another, less calorie-laden alternative. Here's a brief history of the popular plans of the last few decades:

• There have been lots of severely restrictive short-term plans, like the original *Beverly Hills Diet*, which featured platefuls of pineapple and papaya, or the more recent *Cabbage Soup Diet*, or meal-replacement plans with their chocolate and strawberry milkshakes. You get bored on most of these these long before you get vitamin and mineral deficiencies.

- In 1972, Dr Atkins first published his revolutionary idea – that you could lose weight simply and effectively by cutting out carbohydrate foods (bread, potatoes, pasta, and most fruits and vegetables) and focusing on high-fat proteins like meat and cheese. They lost weight but, before long, dieters were suffering from bad breath and constipation, and finding their diets difficult to follow full-time.

- Enter Audrey Eyton with her *F-Plan Diet*, which included plenty of fibre at every meal. The downside soon became apparent when some wag nicknamed it 'The Flatulence Plan'.

- Could the trick lie in food combining, a plan devised by Harvey and Marilyn Diamond, by which you could eat protein and carbohydrates – but not at the same meal? Or did this simply work because dieters were taking in fewer calories?

- Rosemary Conley ruled in the late 1980s and 1990s with her remarkably successful books and videos, which argue that the secret of long-term weight management is cutting right back on fats. The problem was that it's fats that tend to give food flavour and make you feel full up so her dieters often felt starving.

During the 1990s and into the 21st century, new diets seemed to appear every week, many of them addressing the drawbacks of the previous bestseller – and some of them going off at a tangent of their own.

- *The Blood Type Diet* advocates different eating plans according to your blood group because, it argues, each of the four types processes food differently.

- Detox diets are holier-than-thou, cutting out wheat, dairy, alcohol and caffeine to help cleanse the system and boost the metabolism.

- There's been a swing back to ancient eating programmes such as ayurveda and macrobiotics, both of which have received celebrity endorsements but are pretty hard to follow in the modern world.

- Barry Sears introduced one of the more complex systems with the *Zone Diet*, whereby all proteins, carbohydrates and fats had to be eaten in carefully balanced proportions to each other.

These are just some mainstream examples – there are hundreds more less popular types of diet that have come and gone, but none that achieved everything dieters were looking for.

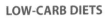

LOW-CARB DIETS

In the early years of the 21st century, there was a huge swing back to Atkins-style diets. The new diet plans still focused on proteins but allowed more non-starchy carbs than the original system. Low-carb breads, cakes and chocolate bars were launched to help keep dieters on track. But the Atkins plan still relied upon an induction phase in which dieters went into a state known as ketosis, cutting carbs so radically that their body burned fat for fuel. Most of the medical establishment was against a diet that restricted foods they considered essential to health, such as fruits and whole grains, and the press debate reached fever pitch, throwing doubt into dieters' minds. In a couple of well-publicised cases, dieters actually died and it was found that they had suffered severe metabolic imbalances as a result of the diet.

The truth was that on the whole low-carb dieters were losing weight, some of them very rapidly, but they still suffered from bad breath and constipation, they didn't feel particularly well – and many of them found that the weight piled back on when they tried to eat normally again. So low-carb systems didn't have all the answers.

However, something interesting definitely seemed to be happening when dieters cut back on carbs. The argument used by the authors of the low-carb diet plans was that carbohydrate foods were broken down rapidly in the digestive system to simple sugars that caused a blood sugar 'spike', and prompted the body to produce excess quantities of the hormone insulin that is responsible for mopping up sugars in the blood. Once the blood sugar level fell again, the dieter would feel cravings for more, and if they ate a lot of carbs they would have peaks and troughs all day long.

High insulin levels signal the body to store more calories as fat, and they also prevent dieters from feeling the cut-off point that tells them they have had enough to eat and are no longer hungry. So they're not good news for anyone.

If maintaining steady blood sugar levels, without any peaks or troughs, was a critical element for weight management, there was a sector of the population who already knew all about it – diabetics.

REGULATING BLOOD SUGAR LEVELS

Diabetes is a disorder in which the pancreas doesn't produce enough insulin, so diabetics are not able to process sugars in their blood and levels can get dangerously high. Type 1 diabetics don't produce any insulin at all, and they require regular injections to keep them alive. Type 2 diabetics don't produce enough insulin for the body's needs, but in most cases they can control their condition with medication, by keeping their weight down and regulating their intake of sugars and carbohydrates to avoid overloading the system.

Both kinds of diabetics have to be very careful about spreading their intake of carbohydrates throughout the day and avoiding sugars. Bingeing on Danish pastries, fizzy drinks and chocolate could induce a diabetic coma. There are special diabetic biscuits and sweets in chemists and health food shops that don't create huge blood sugar rushes, and diabetics are taught to focus on foods that provide slow, steady amounts of energy throughout the day.

Back in the 1980s, scientists realised that not all carbohydrates, starches and sugars produced blood sugar swings because some were broken down more slowly in the digestive system. They began to test different types of carbs and give each a score, according to how quickly they were converted into blood sugar. The list of scores became known as the 'glycaemic index', from the term 'glycogen', the form in which sugars are stored in the body.

- In the glycaemic index (GI for short), pure sugar (glucose) is given a score of 100, the top score.
- High GI foods such as white bread, chips, baked potatoes, doughnuts and easy-cook rice score between 70 and 100.

The Glucose Process

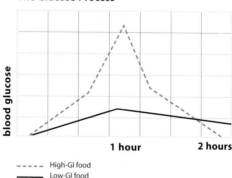

blood glucose

1 hour   2 hours

---- High-GI food
——— Low-GI food

- Medium GI foods, scoring between 55 and 70, include rye crispbreads, bran and fruit cereals, and figs.
- Low GI foods, which are the main ones you are

Some Glycaemic Index Values

Apple juice	40	Mangoes	56
Apples	38	Milk chocolate bar	49
Bagel, plain	72	Milk, whole	27
Baked beans, tinned	48	Muesli	56
Bananas	52	Multi-grain bread	48
Beetroot	64	Mushrooms	<15
Broad beans	79	Oranges	42
Broccoli	<15	Peanuts	15
Cake, sponge	46	Pearl barley	25
Carrots	47	Peas, green	48
Cauliflower	<15	Peppers	<15
Chips	75	Pitta bread, white	57
Couscous	65	Pizza, cheese	60
Crisps	54	Porridge	49
Digestive biscuits	58	Potato, baked	85
Doughnut	76	Rice, brown	55
Gnocchi	67	Soya beans, boiled	16
Grapefruit	25	Soya milk	30
Grapes	46	Spaghetti, white	41
Honey	58	Sugar, white	68
Ice cream	61	Sweetcorn	54
Jam	49	Watermelon	72
Kidney beans, boiled	28	White bread	70
Lentils, green, boiled	29	Yoghurt, low-fat fruit	33

supposed to eat on a GI diet, score less than 55; they include grapefruit, plain yoghurt and red kidney beans.

'GOOD' CARBS VERSUS 'BAD' CARBS

How can you tell whether a food has a low, medium or high GI value? It's not easy without a book like this to hand. In the laboratory, GI testing is a very time-consuming process using human guinea pigs. Each subject eats a carefully measured portion of the test food in question that is known to contain 50g of carbohydrate. Blood samples are then taken from them every 15 minutes for the first hour, then every 30 minutes for the next hour, and their blood sugar level is plotted. The subject's response to the food is compared with their response to consuming 50g of glucose, the reference food. The reference and test food scores are compared for 8 to 10 subjects and the food is awarded a GI score. So, it's not the kind of procedure you can carry out by yourself at home while deciding what to have for dinner.

There are some basic rules you can follow. The simplest way to distinguish between easily absorbed carbs and more slowly absorbed ones is by taste. The sweeter the food, the quicker you're going to get a blood sugar 'rush'. The 'simple' sugars are the fastest carbs to be converted; you'll find them listed on ingredients labels with names like glucose, sucrose (cane or beet sugar), fructose (found in fruits), lactose (milk sugar), galactose, dextrose and maltose. 'Complex' carbs are the slowest to be converted and these include wholegrains, seeds, beans and legumes and some vegetables; they contain a high proportion of dietary fibre which slows down their digestion. Refined processed carbohydrate foods like white bread, cakes and biscuits are quick to convert, mainly because they lack fibre.

The listings in this book split foods into high, medium and low GI categories, because that is the information you will need if you plan to follow a GI diet. However, it is important to understand that the glycaemic index can be misleading, because it doesn't take into account average portion sizes. Jam and carrots have similar GI values, but you would have to eat a lot of raw carrots – 750g or so – for them to have a noticeable effect on your blood sugar, while a dessertspoonful of jam would give you an almost instant blood sugar peak.

Another measure – the Glycaemic Load – gives values according to the effect on blood sugar of a normal portion of the food in question.

Glycaemic Load = (Glycaemic Index value x no. of grams of carb per serving) ÷ 100

Glycaemic Load values are much lower than Glycaemic Index ones:
High GL = 20 or more
Medium GL = 11-19
Low GL = 10 or less

Sugar is a high-GI food, with a score of 100, but if only a teaspoon is consumed it will be low GL, with a score of 4.9. Carrots have a medium GI rating but a low GL count. The key thing to understand is that if you are eating a high-GI food, you can limit the effect on blood sugar by keeping the portion size small.

Here are some other GI rules:
- If you eat a low-GI food with a high-GI one, the overall effect is medium GI.
- Protein and fats slow down the digestion of carbohydrate, so they can reduce the effects of high-GI foods on your blood sugar. Choose a protein, such as a boiled egg, to eat with your morning toast and the

breakfast will have a much lower GI value than if you chose jam or marmalade on toast.

• Fibre slows the absorption of sugars. Apples are low-GI but apple juice is medium-GI, because the fibre in the whole apple reduces the speed at which the fruit sugar is absorbed. Wholegrain products that retain their fibrous content are lower-GI than refined, white products that have had most the fibre stripped away.

• The way you cook a food will affect its GI value. The longer you boil your broccoli, the less fibre it will retain; lightly steaming vegetables and eating them *al dente* means the digestive system has to work harder to break them down and the GI value of the overall meal will be lowered.

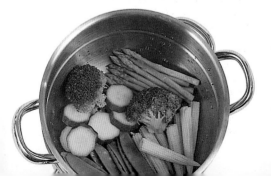

- Some types of starch are harder for the digestive system to break down, so they have lower GI values than other, similar types of food. For example, basmati rice is harder to digest than plain white rice, so it has a lower GI value.

- Acids reduce a food's GI value, so if you squeeze some lemon juice on top of your meal, or sprinkle on a little vinegar, you make it more GI-diet-friendly.

There is advice throughout the listings section of this book on ways to make low-GI meals and snacks.

THE GI FOOD PYRAMID

Foods only have GI values if they contain carbohydrates, but you won't lose weight if you consume excessive amounts of foods that don't contain carbs, or excessive amounts of low-GI foods. GI diets recommend a sensible balance of nutrients and plenty of variety in meals to ensure you consume everything your body needs for good health.

The GI Food Pyramid is a visual demonstration of the proportions of different foods you should consume daily:

Fruit and vegetables – aim to eat at least 5-8 servings a day

Starchy carbohydrates (granary bread, grains, pasta, rice, cereals) – eat 3-6 servings a day
Low-fat milk, yoghurt, cheese – eat 1-3 times a day
Proteins (lean meat, fish, poultry, eggs, beans and nuts) – eat 1-3 times a day
Fats, oils, sweets, white bread and sugary treats – eat only rarely

Don't opt for huge servings. Throughout the listings, calorie, fat, protein and carb counts are given for an average serving, but to save you weighing every time, follow the portion guidelines on pages 22–4.

The GI Food Pyramid

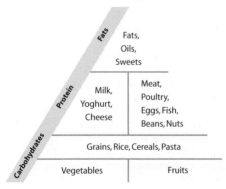

Bakery
A medium slice of bread weighs around 30g.
A 2cm-thick slice of French bread is around 33g.
A standard bagel weighs about 70g.
A muffin in a paper case is about 60g.

Beans and Pulses
Half a teacup of cooked or drained canned beans is about 115g.
A small can of beans in sauce weighs 200g.

Breakfast Cereals
30g of flakes or puffed cereal goes halfway up a normal bowl.
40g high-fibre bran or grapenuts is half a normal bowl, and so is 50g muesli.

Condiments and Sauces
15ml is a level tablespoon and 5 ml is a level teaspoon. Use a medicine spoon as a 5ml measure.

Dairy
15g butter is the quantity you would spread on one slice bread evenly but not thickly.
25g cheese is about the same size as your thumb.
Individual yoghurt pots can vary in size, so check on the side.

Fruit

A tennis ball-sized apple is about 200g (there will be 5 to a kilogram).

A medium banana weighs around 150g.

A half teacup of chopped prepared fruit or berry fruits is about 75g.

Meat and Poultry

75g piece of meat or chicken is about the same size as a pocket pack of tissues.

100g piece is like a pack of cards.

Burgers range from 85g for a skinny one up to 125g for thick ones. A quarterpound burger weighs about 120g.

Rice

2 level tablespoons dry rice will give about 75g when cooked – a mound that's roughly the same size as a woman's fist.

Snacks

25g nuts is roughly the amount a small child could hold in one hand.

25g crisps is a large handful for an adult. Look at the total weight of the pack and judge the portion size from that.

Vegetables

A teacup of salad leaves weighs about 30g.
Half a cup of cooked shredded cabbage is roughly 75g.
Most of the portion sizes given in the listings are
equivalent to half a teacupful, unless otherwise stated.

A simple rule to remember is: when you look at your
dinner plate, around half the space should be filled
with vegetables, a quarter with protein and a quarter
with a low-GI carbohydrate. That is the essence of a
GI diet meal.

WHAT KIND OF PROTEINS AND FATS?

There are two main types of dietary fat – saturated
and unsaturated. Saturated fats tend to come from
animal protein sources: the white fat on cuts of meat,
butter, cream and cheese, lard or dripping.

Unsaturated fats come from vegetable, fish and nut
oils. As most people will be aware, saturated fats got
a bad name because they became associated with
high levels of cholesterol blocking the arteries and
triggering heart disease and strokes.
Atkins diets advocate eating full-fat proteins, because
they make you feel fuller and add flavour to food
while slowing the absorption of carbs. The Atkins
research centres claim that blood tests on people

following their diet shows a reduction in blood pressure and improved cholesterol levels. However, most medical professionals and certainly the vast majority of heart specialists give the opposite advice – that you should choose low-fat or fat-free dairy products and lean meats – and most GI diets go along with the low-fat approach.

Proteins are essential for good health, providing the materials from which bones, muscles, hair, nails, blood, enzymes and hormones are created. They aren't just found in meat, fish, cheese and eggs, though; vegetable proteins include soya products like tofu, beans and pulses, brown rice, broccoli, bananas and many other fruits and vegetables. Adults only need 60g of protein a day, but most of us eat a lot more. We also need some fats in our diet, even when we are trying to lose weight, because important nutrients are supplied by 'good' fats. Here are the fats to opt for and the ones to avoid:

- Monounsaturated fats, found in olive and rapeseed oil, walnuts and almonds, have beneficial effects on the heart.

- Omega 3 fats, found in oily fishes like salmon, mackerel and herring, flaxseed oils, wheatgerm and soya beans, help to thin the blood and are crucial for brain function.

- Polyunsaturated fats, found in vegetable and corn oils, don't have the health benefits of mono-unsaturated fats but, like most fats, they contain 135 calories per tablespoonful, so should be used sparingly when you're trying to lose weight.

- Saturated fats include all the animal fats, plus coconut and palm oils, which are often found in biscuits and snacks. Try to avoid eating them too frequently.

- Hydrogenated or trans fats are the worst kind, linked to high cholesterol levels and increased heart disease risk. You'll find them in various kinds of ready-made meals, biscuits and cakes, breads and spreads, vegetable shortening, peanut butter, pastries, margarines and fast foods.

VITAMINS AND MINERALS

On paper, GI diets are better for you than low-carb/high-protein diets, because they don't try to cut out or restrict any whole food group. However, it's down to each individual to make sure they eat a wide enough range of foods to get all the vitamins and minerals they need for good health. One tip is to make sure all the portions of fruits and vegetables you eat in a day are different colours: dark green kale, yellow corn, red peppers, orange carrots, translucent onions, pale green avocados, pale yellow melon, purple sprouting broccoli, blackberries, apricots, blueberries, bananas. Your plate will look more attractive, and you will be getting different types of micronutrient from each.

Look through the vitamins and minerals chart that follows and make sure you eat foods containing each of them on a daily – or at least weekly – basis. If this is going to be difficult, you might consider taking a supplement, but never exceed the Recommended Daily Dose (RDA) on the pack because some can be dangerous in high doses.

VITAMINS AND MINERALS

Vitamin A Eggs, butter, fish oils, dark green and yellow fruits and vegetables, liver.
Essential for: strong bones, good eyesight, healthy skin, healing.

Vitamin B1 (*Thiamine*): Plant and animal foods, especially wholegrain products, brown rice, seafood and beans.
Essential for: growth, nerve function, conversion of blood sugar into energy.

Vitamin B2 (*Riboflavin*): Milk and dairy produce, green leafy vegetables, liver, kidneys, yeast.
Essential for: cell growth and reproduction, energy production.

Vitamin B3 (*Niacin*): Meats, fish and poultry, wholegrains, peanuts and avocados.
Essential for: digestion, energy, the nervous system.

Vitamin B5 (*Pantothenic acid*): Organ meats, fish, eggs, chicken, nuts and wholegrain cereals.
Essential for: strengthening immunity and fighting infections, healing wounds.

Vitamin B6 (*Pyridoxine*): Meat, eggs, wholegrains, yeast, cabbage, melon, molasses.
Essential for: the production of new cells, a healthy immune system, production of antibodies and white blood cells.

Vitamin B12 (*Cyanocolbalamin*): Fish, dairy produce, beef, pork, lamb, organ meats, eggs and milk.
Essential for: energy and concentration, production of red blood cells, growth in children.

Vitamin C: Fresh fruit and vegetables, potatoes, leafy herbs and berries.
Essential for: healthy skin, bones, muscles, healing, eyesight and protection from viruses.

Vitamin D: Milk and dairy produce, eggs, fatty fish.
Essential for: healthy teeth and bones, vital for growth.

Vitamin E: Nuts, seeds, eggs, milk, wholegrains, leafy vegetables, avocados and soya. *Essential for:* absorption of iron and essential fatty acids, slowing the ageing process, increasing fertility.

Vitamin K: Green vegetables, milk products, apricots, wholegrains, cod liver oil. *Essential for:* blood clotting.

Calcium: Dairy produce, leafy green vegetables, salmon, nuts, root vegetables, tofu. *Essential for:* strong bones and teeth, hormones and muscles, blood clotting and the regulation of blood pressure.

Iron: Liver, kidney, cocoa powder, dark chocolate, shellfish, pulses, dark green vegetables, egg yolks, red meat, beans, molasses. *Essential for:* supply of oxygen to the cells and healthy immune system.

Magnesium: Brown rice, soya beans, nuts, wholegrains, bitter chocolate, legumes. *Essential for:* transmission of nerve impulses, development of bones, growth and repair of cells.

Potassium: Avocados, leafy green vegetables, bananas, fruit and vegetable juices, potatoes and nuts. *Essential for:* maintaining

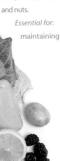

water balance, nerve and muscle function.

Chromium: Liver, whole grains, meat and cheese, brewer's yeast, mushrooms, egg yolk.

Essential for: stimulating insulin. Chromium also governs the 'glucose tolerance factor' which is often not working properly in failed dieters.

Iodine: Fish and seafood, pineapple, dairy produce, raisins.

Essential for: keeping hair, skin, nails and teeth healthy.

Folic acid: Fruit, green leafy vegetables, nuts, pulses, yeast extracts.

Essential for: production of new cells (working with vitamin B12) and is especially important during pregnancy to prevent birth defects.

READING LABELS

You won't find GI values listed on the packaging of many foods in the UK, although Tesco have introduced a 'Low-GI' logo for their own-brand foods. However, reading the ingredients labels and bearing in mind the basic GI rules outlined above should help you to make an informed decision about which foods are low GI. Ingredients are listed on food packaging in descending order of volume, so if sugars or fats are near the beginning, alarm bells should be ringing.

- Watch out for sugar in all its guises: it might be labelled glucose, sucrose, invertase, fructose, lactose, galactose, maltose, dextrose or honey.

- You will probably recognise the names for fats. Watch out for hydrogenated, partially hydrogenated or trans fats, and give them a wide berth.

- Long lists of E numbers, artificial colours and flavours are always a turn-off.

Under Nutrition Information, look for the following:
- Calorie count should be given per portion, per pack and/or per 100g or 100ml. Note that manufacturers' portion sizes can be extremely small and it can be easy to eat twice as much as they estimate. Don't overlook calories on a low-GI diet – you will put on weight if you are consuming more calories a day than you are burning off through exercise, regardless of whether they are 'low-GI' calories.

- Carbohydrates will be listed, and the label will probably indicate how much of the carb total is made up of sugars.

- Fat content will be given as total fat, then the percentage of saturates, monounsaturates and polyunsaturates will be given.

- Choose high-fibre products; aim for more than 5g fibre per 100g serving.

- Are there vitamins and minerals listed? It should give the percentage of the Recommended Daily Allowance supplied by an average portion or 100g/100ml.

Nutrition flashes on the front of packaging can be misleading:

- The term 'fat-free' can be applied to foods containing less than 0.15g fat per 100g. However, the term '90% fat-free' means that the product actually has 10% fat.

- 'Virtually fat-free' means the food contains less than 0.3g fat per 100g. 'Low-fat' means the food must contain 3g or fewer of fat per 100g. 'Reduced fat' means the food contains 25% less fat than the standard equivalent product.

- 'No added sugar' means that no sugar has been added during processing or manufacture but it does not necessarily mean that the food is low in sugar. 'Unsweetened' means that no sugar or sweetener has been added.

- There is no legal definition of the term 'reduced salt' but the Food Standards Agency recommends that food with this label should contain 25% less salt or sodium than an equivalent product.

• 'Rich source of...' a vitamin or mineral means the product must contain 50% of the RDA in a typical serving. If it says 'Source of...' then a serving must contain at least 17% RDA.

HOW MUCH WEIGHT DO YOU NEED TO LOSE?

Before you start any weight-loss diet, you should have an idea of what would be a healthy weight for you. There's no point in choosing unrealistic goals. If you have a naturally rounded figure, you will make yourself ill trying to diet down to stick-insect size proportions. If you have a large frame, you will never shrink to a small frame no matter how little you eat. Everyone is born with a genetically predisposed natural weight range. If you consistently eat too much and don't exercise, your weight will exceed this range. If you diet down to a weight below your natural range, you will find it hard to maintain.

Height and weight charts, such as the one on pages 34-5, give an ideal weight for your height. However, these are just approximations that reflect cultural averages. Two people of the same height and build can have completely different weights and yet both be healthy. Muscle weighs more than fat, so someone who exercises regularly might weigh more than

Tables for Standard Body Weight

Men

Height m (ft)	Small Frame kg (lbs)	Medium Frame kg (lbs)	Large Frame kg (lbs)
1.55 (5'1")	49–59 (107–130)	51–61 (113–134)	55–64 (121–140)
1.57 (5'2")	50–60 (110–132)	53–63 (116–138)	56–65 (124–144)
1.60 (5'3")	51–61 (113–134)	54–64 (119–140)	58–68 (127–150)
1.63 (5'4")	53–61 (116–135)	55–65 (122–142)	59–70 (131–154)
1.65 (5'5")	54–62 (119–137)	57–66 (125–146)	60–72 (133–159)
1.68 (5'6")	56–64 (123–140)	59–68 (129–149)	62–74 (137–163)
1.70 (5'7")	58–65 (127–143)	60–69 (133–152)	64–76 (142–167)
1.73 (5'8")	60–66 (131–145)	62–71 (137–155)	66–78 (146–171)
1.75 (5'9")	61–68 (135–149)	64–72 (141–158)	68–80 (150–175)
1.78 (5'10")	63–69 (139–152)	66–73 (145–161)	70–81 (154–179)
1.80 (5'11")	65–70 (143–155)	68–75 (149–165)	72–83 (159–183)
1.83 (6')	67–72 (147–159)	70–77 (153–169)	74–85 (163–187)
1.85 (6'1")	69–75 (151–165)	71–80 (157–175)	76–86 (167–189)
1.88 (6'2")	70–76 (155–168)	73–81 (161–179)	78–89 (171–197)
1.90 (6'3")	72–79 (157–173)	75–84 (166–185)	80–92 (176–202)

Women

Height m (ft)	Small Frame kg (lbs)	Medium Frame kg (lbs)	Large Frame kg (lbs)
1.47 (4'10")	41–49 (91–108)	43–52 (95–115)	47–54 (103–119)
1.50 (4'11")	42–51 (93–112)	44–55 (98–121)	48–57 (106–125)
1.52 (5')	44–52 (96–115)	46–57 (101–124)	49–58 (109–128)
1.55 (5'1")	45–54 (99–118)	47–58 (104–127)	51–59 (112–131)
1.57 (5'2")	46–55 (102–121)	49–60 (107–132)	52–61 (115–135)
1.60 (5'3")	48–56 (105–124)	50–62 (110–135)	54–63 (118–138)
1.63 (5'4")	49–58 (108–127)	51–63 (113–138)	55–65 (122–142)
1.65 (5'5")	50–59 (111–130)	53–64 (117–141)	57–66 (126–145)
1.68 (5'6")	52–60 (115–133)	55–66 (121–144)	59–67 (130–148)
1.70 (5'7")	54–62 (119–136)	57–67 (125–147)	61–69 (134–151)
1.73 (5'8")	56–63 (123–139)	58–68 (128–150)	62–71 (137–155)
1.75 (5'9")	58–64 (127–142)	60–69 (133–153)	64–73 (141–159)
1.78 (5'10")	59–66 (131–145)	62–71 (137–156)	66–75 (146–165)
1.80 (5'11")	61–68 (135–148)	64–72 (141–159)	68–77 (150–170)
1.83 (6')	63–69 (138–151)	65–74 (143–163)	69–79 (153–173)

someone of the same height who is sedentary. This is why doctors are now more likely to calculate your body mass index (BMI) to see whether you are overweight or not. BMI is a height to weight formula that gives a good approximation of total body fat. To find your BMI, divide your weight in kilograms by the square of your height in metres:

weight ÷ (height x height)

For example, if you are 1.75m tall and weigh 64kg:

1.75 x 1.75 = 3.06
64 ÷ 3.06 = 20.91

Check your total against the list below to see if you fall into an average range.

less than 15	emaciated
15–19	underweight
19–25	average
25–30	overweight
30–40	obese

If your BMI is in the emaciated or obese range, you should consult your doctor for advice, as you could be seriously endangering your health.

WAIST MEASUREMENT

Waist measurements of more than 100cm (40 inches) for men and more than 88cm (35 inches) for women are linked with all kinds of health risks, particularly an increased risk of heart disease. Another indicator that doctors use is your waist to hip ratio:

waist measurement ÷ hip measurement = ?

Above 1.0 for men and 0.85 for women puts you into an at-risk category.

Your ideal weight is the one at which you feel healthy, energetic and comfortable. Once you reach an 'average' BMI score, then you are a healthy weight. How much do you think you want to lose? What BMI rating would this give for your height? So how much do you need to lose to take you down into an average BMI category? This is a sensible target to adopt.

Don't try to lose more than a kilogram a week, or you will be likely to put it all back on again as soon as you stop dieting. Slow and steady is the best plan. If you want to lose 10 kilos, allow at least three months; for 20 kilos, allow at least 6 months; and for 40 kilos, give yourself a year. Experts say that a realistic target is to lose between 5 and 10% of your starting body weight within 6 months.

Consult a doctor before starting a weight-loss programme if any of the following apply to you:
- You have a chronic condition such as coronary heart disease, or have had a stroke
- You take any medication
- You are pregnant
- You are over 40 years old and have more than 5 kilos to lose
- You are planning to start an exercise programme as well, but haven't exercised for years.

EXERCISE

Most weight-loss experts agree that the first thing you should do on a weight-loss plan is to increase your level of physical activity. Muscle burns more calories than fat, so once you increase the amount of muscle in your body, you will be burning off more energy even when you are sitting watching television.

No matter what kind of diet you decide to follow, calories still count. To lose half a kilo per week, you need to reduce your calorie intake by 500 kcal a day or 3500 per week. However, a one-hour aerobics class might burn off around 400 kcal; half an hour of jogging could burn 250 kcal, and 15 minutes of brisk walking could burn 75 kcal. This means that if you are exercising, you won't need to cut back what you eat quite so drastically!

There is also evidence that exercise helps to keep your blood sugar levels steady by triggering the release of hormones that regulate them. And it stimulates the release of endorphins, which make you feel good and relieve stress and depression.

WHY CHOOSE THE GI DIET?

The medical establishment generally approves of GI diets because they are not extreme crash diets that exclude important food groups. Instead they should be seen as an eating plan that you can follow for life. Making your blood sugar levels steadier means that you shouldn't suffer sugar cravings or feel hungry, yet there's no need to weigh foods and count calories, net carbs, points or grams of fat, as for other diets.

Eating low-GI carbs isn't the whole story, however. You are advised to opt for low-fat protein sources, which will keep your doctor happy, and you should also avoid heavily processed foods with lots of artificial additives, which would make it very hard to work out the GI value. Most fruits and vegetables are allowed, and you are encouraged to eat healthy fats like fish oils, nuts and seeds.

GI diets will suit vegetarians and vegans, with their emphasis on vegetables and pulses. They will be easy to follow for those who have to dine out frequently because there are plenty of low-GI choices in almost every kind of restaurant (see pages 217–31). It's not complex to follow, so will suit those who don't have much time on their hands.

Low-GI foods tend to be low-calorie as well but if you eat massive quantities of them, you will still gain weight. The only downside of the GI plan is that it requires you to be self-disciplined about your portion sizes and make sure you get a good-enough range of nutrients. It makes sense to follow one of the detailed plans on the market until you have enough under-standing of how it works to devise your own meals and recipes. Here's a look at four of the most popular.

RICK GALLOP – THE GI DIET

Rick Gallop has been the President of the Heart and Stroke Foundation of Ontario, Canada for more than 20 years. He began investigating GI diets after a back injury meant he could no longer exercise and he put on 9kg (20lb). After trying several leading diets to no avail, he developed his own, based on low GI foods. He spent many years honing the diet to make it easy to understand and to follow. His books list foods in three columns: red for high GI, yellow for medium GI and green for Low GI.

Gallop advises that you choose a target weight that will give you a body mass index of between 22 and 24. He suggests that you visualise the weight you want to lose by putting an equivalent weight in bags of sugar in a rucksack and carrying it around for half a day. The feeling of freedom after you take that weight off your back will help to motivate you to lose the kilos you need to.

Before you start Phase 1 of the diet, he suggests that you record all your vital statis-tics. Throughout this phase, you will weigh yourself every day. You are told to clear all red and yellow list foods from your storecupboard and fridge and shop for foods on the green list. The permitted

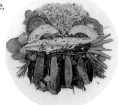

THE TEN GOLDEN RULES FOR RICK GALLOP'S GI DIET ARE:

Eat three meals and three snacks every day.

In Phase 1 eat only low GI foods.

Restrict portion sizes of meat, pasta and rice.

Keep the correct ratio of carbs, protein and fat.

Eat three times as many fruits and vegetables than normal.

Drink plenty of fluid, preferably water.

Exercise for 30 minutes a day.

Find a friend for mutual support.

Set realistic goals.

Don't look on the regime as a diet but more as a way of living.

foods are low-calorie, low-fat and high fibre, and include plenty of fruits and vegetables.

The GI Diet is not an all-you-can-eat diet. During Phase 1, portions of meat and fish should weigh no more than 100g; the dry weight of a portion of pasta should be 40g and rice should be 50g. You are advised to eat three meals and up to three snacks a day, but are only allowed foods from the low-GI column. You follow Phase 1 until you reach your target weight, and then switch to Phase 2, which will help you maintain it. You can gradually add back medium-GI foods and increase your calorie intake, but you are advised to get plenty of exercise so that you are expending as much energy as you eat and keep weighing yourself to make sure the weight doesn't creep back on.

Phase 1 Sample Menus
Breakfast choices
Porridge or 2-egg-white omelette or bran cereal with fresh fruit and cottage cheese

Lunch choices
Vegetable Salad, dressed with low-fat vinaigrette and 115g (4oz) low-fat protein or Pasta Salad Lunch or an Open Sandwich

Dinner choices
Chicken Curry or Baked Fish on a bed of Leeks and Onions or Meat Loaf.

Snack choices
Eat three a day. Try a high-protein nutrition bar, low-fat cottage cheese and raw vegetables, fruit yoghurt or fresh fruit.

THE GI DIET PHASE 1

Foods to enjoy

Oat and high-fibre cereals

Fruit and fruit juice, but not bananas or dates

Salads and seasonal vegetables

Skinless chicken and turkey breast

Oily fish

Nuts

Cottage cheese

Basmati rice

Foods to avoid

Butter

Bacon

Whole eggs (just use the white)

Coffee and tea, unless decaffeinated

Any desserts

Chips

Baguettes

Alcohol

Effectiveness

If you keep to the portion sizes Gallop recommends and stick to green-light foods, you will lose weight steadily on this diet. The focus on foods that are low-

PHASE 2
Foods to reintroduce
Lean bacon
Bananas (occasionally)
Caffeinated drinks
Sweetcorn cobs
Glass of wine with dinner
Low-fat icecream
Pasta
Boiled potatoes
Foods to avoid or eat rarely
Large portions of any food
Fried or mashed potato
Beer
Chocolate
Sugar-coated breakfast cereal
Cakes and desserts
Biscuits
Fish in breadcrumbs or batter

calorie as well as low-GI means that weight is more likely to stay off long-term. The colour coding makes the choices easy to follow and recipe ideas are interesting. The only drawback is that the rest of the family might complain about you throwing out all medium- and high-GI foods, and not stocking banned foods such as butter. Gallup also advocates the use of artificial sweeteners like aspartame, about which many nutritionists have concerns.

AZMINA GOVINDJI AND NINA PUDDEFOOT – THE GI PLAN

Govindji used to be a dietician for Diabetes UK and Puddefoot is a life development coach. Their plan is based on standard low-GI diet guidelines but foods have been given point values known as 'GIPs'. During the 'start-it' phase, for the first two weeks of the diet, women are allowed 17 points a day and men 22. In week 3, you enter the 'lose-it' phase and points allowances rise to 20 for women and 25 for men.

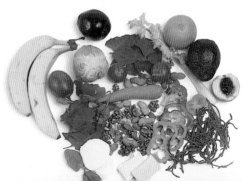

THE GI PLAN	
Foods to enjoy	**Foods to avoid or eat rarely**
Fresh fruit	Cornflakes
Fresh and frozen vegetables	White bread
Bran and oat breakfast cereals	Sweet fizzy drinks
Granary and wholemeal bread	Chips or mashed potato
Brown and basmati rice	Fatty meat
Dried beans and lentils	Pastries and cakes
Lean meat and poultry	Meat pies
Olive and rapeseed oil and spray oil	Biscuits
Water – still and sparkling	Rice cakes
Plain pasta	Canned fruit in syrup
Plain low-fat yoghurt	Jasmine rice
Fish	Dried dates
Meat substitutes like Quorn®	Confectionery

There are plenty of meal and recipe ideas, all of them listing their points value, and you are told to eat three meals and three snacks spread evenly throughout the day.

You remain on the 'lose-it' phase until you reach your target weight, when you switch to a 'Keep-it' phase with a points allowance of 23 or more for women and 28 or more for men. You should aim to lose no more than a kilo per week.

Sample menus
Breakfast choices
Branflakes and an apple
Granary bread with scrambled egg
Wholemeal bread with peanut butter and half a cantaloupe melon

Lunch choices
Chicken Tortilla with salad and diet yoghurt
Jacket potato with tuna and sweetcorn and a packet of soup
Baguette with prawns and salad and a pear

Dinner choices
Turkey Stroganoff with rice and tomato salad, plus orange juice

Salmon Steaks in Garlic Balsamic with Fettucine and steamed asparagus tips, followed by canned peaches in juice

Vegetarian options include garlic mushrooms or cabbage with fennel seeds or roasted vegetables

Snack choices

Cereal bar

Almonds

Packet of tomato soup

Another aspect of the book is the motivational advice, lifestyle hints and affirmations you are supposed to repeat, such as 'Every day, in every way, I feel amazing' and 'Surround yourself with joyful people'. Some may find these helpful, while others could find them irritating.

Effectiveness

If you adhere to your points allowance, you would lose weight on this diet. However, it could be tricky to eat out since you wouldn't be able to judge the points value of any but very plain foods. The menu plans are nutritionally sound and most dieters should find they don't go hungry, but following them exactly could be very restrictive on a day-to-day level and may not fit in with family life.

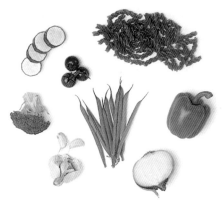

JENNIE BRAND-MILLER –
THE LOW GI DIET

Brand-Miller is Professor of Human Nutrition at the University of Sydney and she has been researching GI values and publishing books and GI listings for 25 years now. *The Low-GI Diet* takes a scientific approach, explaining how digestion and the insulin response work before recommending that you follow a 12-week action plan to lose weight. You work out your 'energy level', take your weight and are then allotted a number of servings of different nutrients each day, based on your gender.

Each week you are given a food goal, an exercise goal, an activity goal and 'food for thought'. There are detailed exercise and menu plans, and you have to fill out daily questionnaires and note everything you eat. Weight-loss advice includes:

· Eat seven or more servings of fruit and vegetables a day
· Eat low-GI breads and cereals
· Eat more beans, including soybeans, chickpeas and lentils
· Eat nuts regularly
· Eat more fish and seafood
· Eat lean red meat, poultry and eggs
· Eat low-fat dairy products

Once you reach your target weight, you should maintain it by following some basic rules:
· Don't skip meals
· Eat a good breakfast
· Eat three or four times a day
· Limit TV viewing to 12 hours a week
· Choose low-GI carbs at every meal
· Eat lean protein at every meal.
· Don't skimp on fats – just choose healthy ones.
· Eat seven servings of vegetables and fruit every day.
· Exercise for 30–60 minutes six out of seven days.
· On the seventh day, relax and enjoy.

THE LOW GI DIET	
Foods to enjoy	**Foods to avoid or eat rarely**
Vegetables	Confectionery
Sweet potato	Biscuits
All fruits, especially berry fruits	Crisps
Granary and stone-ground bread	Large portions of any food
Fruit loaf	Cornflakes and corn pasta
Bulgur wheat	White bread
Oats	Canned spaghetti
Durum wheat pasta	Short-grain rice
Basmati rice	Fatty meat
Beans and soya beans	
Nuts and nut butter	
Oily fish	
Plain yoghurt	

Sample menus
Breakfast choices
Toasted wholegrain bread with ricotta cheese and fruit jam
Poached egg with smoked salmon and spinach on wholegrain toast
A nut and seed bar and an apple

Lunch choices
Tortilla wrap with chicken, lettuce, tomato, cucumber and salsa
Roast beef sandwich on wholegrain bread with salad and mustard
Lean ham, pineapple and grated light cheese on toasted mixed grain muffin

Dinner choices
Pan-fried pork with spinach, onion and new potatoes
Mushroom and vegetable stir fry
Grilled fish fillet with a handful of crisps and a rocket salad

Snack choices
Low-fat fruit yoghurt
Banana
Handful of pistachio nuts in their shells

Effectiveness

The advice and listings in Brand-Miller's book are comprehensive, but she focuses on foods that are available in the Australian and US markets which may not have exact equivalents here. The plan itself is quite strict and would require a lot of planning and preparation, which might not suit those who are pressed for time. There aren't many vegetarian options. However, anyone who followed the plan to the letter would certainly lose weight, and the long-term eating plans are healthy and nutritionally sound.

ANTONY WORRALL THOMPSON'S GI DIET

When the well-known chef Antony Worrall Thompson was diagnosed with Syndrome X, a precursor of type 2 diabetes, he decided to try and prevent diabetes developing by following the GI diet and taking more exercise. In his book, there are 120 low-GI recipes you can try, as well as cooking tips and some useful general advice on nutrition.

You should still enjoy your food when following this diet, he explains, and you will feel full because low-GI foods take longer to digest than those with higher GI values.

ANTONY WORRALL THOMPSON'S GI DIET	
Foods to enjoy	**Foods to avoid or eat rarely**
Stir-fries with lots of vegetables, beans and peas	Biscuits
	Easy-cook white rice
Basmati rice	Liver
Fruit salads	Egg yolks
Dried fruit compôtes	Shellfish
Fruit crumbles made with oats	Sweet drinks
	Pastry dishes
Grilled lean bacon	Creamy sauces
Poached egg	Fish in batter
Baked fish	
Lentil soup	
New potatoes cooked in their skins	
Pitta breads filled with salad	
Baked beans on toast	

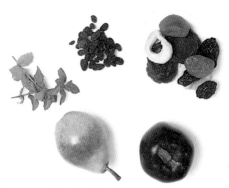

Some specific tips include:
- Make risotto with basmati rice instead of the more traditional arborio
- Eat oat biscuits with cheese instead of wheaten biscuits
- Serve curry with chickpeas or lentils instead of rice
- Include oats in fruit crumble toppings
- Make fruit salads with fresh and dried fruits

He stresses that the diet should not be obsessive but the aim should be to make concessions which will help to reduce or replace the GI content of carbs. This is not a strictly regimented diet, so it would suit those who like to have the freedom to eat out, rather than weighing and preparing set meals three times a day.

Sample menus
Breakfast choices
Egg-white omelette
Porridge with berry fruits
Banana smoothie

Lunch choices
Smoked salmon and cottage cheese sandwich and
fruit
Roast chicken with sweet potatoes
Leek and pea soup

Dinner choices
Thai fishcakes with salad
Barley and goats' cheese soufflé
Pan-fried mullet with olives and tomatoes

Snack choices
Soda bread roll
One slice orange and almond cake
Scotch pancakes and honey

Effectiveness
You would have to be disciplined in the way you followed the diet and avoid excessive portion sizes, but
the recipes are delicious, as you would expect, and
should keep the family and non-dieters happy as well.

HOW TO USE THIS BOOK

The foods in this book are grouped into categories –
Bakery, Biscuits, Condiments and Sauces, etc. – and
listed in alphabetical order in the left-hand column of
each page, together with portion sizes and cooking
methods, where applicable. The emphasis is on whole
foods, since these are the mainstay of all the GI diets.

The portion sizes given are 'average' ones that you
might eat in a single serving, such as one medium
apple, or 100g of chicken breast. We have also used
cup measurements where they are helpful, because
it's easier to visualise a cup of salad than to weigh
out a specific weight of lettuce leaves, especially if
you are eating in a restaurant. Note: think of a
teacup-full rather than a huge mug!

The first column in the listings section gives a red,
yellow or green rating to each food, according to
whether it is High-GI (more than 70), Medium-GI (55
to 70) or Low-GI (under 55). If the first column is
blank, it means the food in question does not have a
GI value. If your diet only allows you to eat low-GI
foods, you should choose those that have a green
rating, or no rating at all. In a long-term eating plan,
you just have to avoid the red-rated foods.

The second column gives the carbohydrate content of the portion in grams; the third lists its fibre content; the fourth column from the left gives the calorie count, in kilocalories, and the fifth and sixth give protein and fat counts in grams.

These portion sizes may not accord with the portion sizes your diet recommends or that you wish to eat. To find the values for a 40g piece of chicken breast, you would have to divide the figures given by 100 and multiply by 40. Read the weights on packaging of any ready-prepared food as portion sizes will vary from product to product.

Note that values are given for cooked products rather than raw. Pasta, rice and pulses swell up to approximately three times their weight when cooked, but food packaging often gives the values for their dry weight.

Values for unbranded foods have been obtained from *The Composition of Foods* (5th edition, 1991 and 6th summary edition, 2002) and *Vegetables, Herbs and Spices* (supplement, 1991), and have been repro- duced by permission of Controller of Her Majesty's Stationery Office. Asda kindly supplied additional information.

The publishers are grateful to all manufacturers who gave information on their products. If you cannot find a particular food here, you can obtain much fuller listings of nutrient counts in branded foods from *Collins Gem Calorie Counter* and *Collins Gem Carb Counter*.

CONVERSION CHART

Metric to imperial
100 grams (g) = 3.53 ounces (oz)
1 kilogram (kg) = 2.2 pounds (lb)
100 millilitres (ml) = 3.38 fluid ounces (fl oz)
1 litre = 1.76 pints

Imperial to metric
1 ounce (oz) = 28.35 grams (g)
1 pound (lb) = 453.60 grams (g)
1 stone (st) = 6.35 kilograms (kg)
1 fluid ounce (fl oz) = 29.57 millilitres (ml)
1 pint = 0.568 litres (l)

Abbreviations used in the listings
g	gram
kcal	kilocalorie
ml	millilitre
n/a	figures not available
—	none

The Listings

BAKERY

Most types of bread don't have a low-GI score because they are made from refined white flour with the fibre stripped out. Ciabatta, baguettes and all kinds of white bread break down into blood glucose very rapidly. On a GI diet, look out for stoneground, granary or wholemeal breads, especially those that are sprinkled with seeds and grains. Pumpernickel, rye and sourdough breads are all low-GI. Some package descriptions can be misleading – multigrain doesn't necessarily mean that the bread is unrefined. When in doubt, compare the fibre counts per slice.

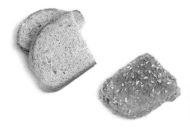

TIP: If you want a sandwich, opt for a lean protein and salad filling and hold the mayonnaise. Salmon, chicken, hummus, avocado, eggs and low-fat cheese will all lower the GI count of your sandwich.

Food type	GI	Carb (g)	Fibre (g)	Cal (kcal)	Pro (g)	Fat (g)
Bread						
Brown, 1 slice	●	13.3	1.8	65	2.6	0.6
Brown, toasted, 1 slice	●	17.0	2.1	82	3.1	0.6
Chapattis:						
made with fat, each (50g)	●	24.1	–	164	4	6.5
made without fat, each (50g)	●	21.8	–	101	3.6	0.5
Ciabatta, 1 slice	●	15	0.7	81	3.1	1.2
Currant loaf, 1 slice	●	15.2	1.3	87	2.2	1.1
French stick, 1 slice (2cm thick)	●	18.4	1.7	90	3.2	0.9
Garlic bread, pre-packed, frozen, 1 slice	●	13.5	–	110	2.3	5.5
Granary, 1 slice	◐	13.9	1.9	70	2.8	0.8
High-bran, 1 slice	◔	10.1	2.4	64	3.9	0.8
Malt, 1 slice	◔	17.1	2.0	80	2.5	0.7
Naan, plain, half	●	35.0	2.0	209	5.5	5.2
Oatmeal, 1 slice	◐	12.4	1.1	70	2.4	1.2
Pitta bread, white, medium:	◔	28.9	1.1	133	4.6	0.6
white with sesame	◔	24	1.5	131	4.8	1.8
wholewheat	◔	20.5	3.1	114	5.4	1.2
Pitta bread, 2 mini (10g each)	◔	11.4	0.7	52	1.7	0.3
Pumpernickel, 1 slice	◐	14.1	1.7	68	2.3	0.5
Rye, 1 slice	◐	13.7	1.7	66	2.4	0.5
Sourdough, 1 slice	◐	14.7	0.9	78	2.5	0.9
Stoneground wholemeal, 1 slice	●	11.8	2.2	65	2.9	0.7

Food type	GI	Carb (g)	Fibre (g)	Cal (kcal)	Pro (g)	Fat (g)
Wheatgerm, 1 slice	●	12.5	1.5	64	2.8	0.6
White, 1 slice	●	14.8	1.2	71	2.5	0.6
White, fried in oil/lard, 1 slice	●	14.5	1.2	151	2.4	9.6
White, toasted, 1 slice	●	17.1	1.4	80	2.8	0.5
Wholemeal, 1 slice	●	12.5	2.2	65	2.8	0.8
Rolls						
Bagels, each (70g):	●	37.2	1.5	192	7.8	1.0
onion bagels	●	37.7	1.5	192	7.8	1.1
sesame bagels	●	36.9	1.5	190	7.9	1.3
cinnamon & raisin	●	39.2	1.5	197	7.4	1.3
Baps, white, each (60g)	●	26.2	1.6	141	5.9	2.6
Brown, crusty, each (60g)	●	30.2	4.3	153	6.2	1.7
Brown, soft, each (60g)	●	31.1	3.8	161	6	2.3
Hamburger bun, each (60g)	●	29.3	0.9	158	5.5	3
White, crusty, each (60g)	●	34.6	2.6	168	6.5	2.6
White, soft, each (60g)	●	31.0	2.3	161	5.5	2.5
Wholemeal, each (60g)	●	29.0	5.3	145	5.4	1.7
Taco shells, each (30g)	●	18.2	–	146	2.2	13.8
Tortillas, each (30g):						
corn	●	13.2	–	95	3.0	3.3
flour	●	10.3	–	103	3.0	2.0

TIP: There are many alternatives to sandwiches for a working lunch in the office. See page 232 for some low-GI packed lunch suggestions.

Food type	GI	Carb (g)	Fibre (g)	Cal (kcal)	Pro (g)	Fat (g)
Tea Breads, Buns, Pastries						
Brioche, each (60g)	●	35.0	–	209	4.9	5.6
Chelsea bun, each (70g)	●	39.3	1.2	256	5.4	9.8
Croissant, each (70g)	●	26.8	1.8	252	5.8	14
Crumpet, each (50g)	◐	17.9	–	89	3.6	0.4
Currant bun, each (70g)	●	36.9	–	207	5	4.6
Danish pastry, each (70g)	●	35.9	1.1	262	4	12.6
Doughnut, each (70g):						
jam	●	34.2	–	235	3.9	10.5
ring	●	33	–	278	4.3	15.4
Eccles cake, each (60g)	●	35.6	1.0	285	2.3	15.6
Fruit loaf, slice (70g)	◐	42.5	–	217	5.3	2.9
Hot cross bun, each (70g)	●	40.9	1.2	217	5.3	4.8
Muffin, each (70g):						
English	◐	32.7	1.6	167	6.3	1.2
blueberry	●	34.9	0.8	300	3	0.8
Potato scone, each (60g)	●	25.2	2.6	124	2.8	1.3
Raisin and cinnamon loaf, slice (70g)	◐	37	2.9	193	5.2	2.7
Scone, each (60g):						
fruit	◐	31.7	–	190	4.4	5.9

TIP: Tea breads like fruit loaf or raisin and cinnamon loaf contain less sugar than cakes. Cut a thin slice and eat without butter when you feel a cake moment coming on.

Food type	GI	Carb (g)	Fibre (g)	Cal (kcal)	Pro (g)	Fat (g)
Scones contd:						
plain	●	32.2	1.0	218	4.3	8.9
wholemeal	●	25.9	3.1	196	5.2	8.4
Scotch pancake, each (60g)	●	26.2	0.8	175	3.5	7.2
Cakes and Cream Cakes						
Almond slice (50g bar)	●	29.3	0.8	191	3.4	6.5
Apple Danish (50g bar)	●	21.4	0.5	120	2.1	12
Bakewell slice (50g)	●	29.7	0.5	218	1.9	10
Banana cake, slice (75g)	●	41.9	0.5	260	2.4	6
Battenburg, slice (75g)	●	52.7	0.9	323	5.3	6.5
Brownies, chocolate, each (75g)	●	36.7	1	311	3.9	15.7
Caramel shortcake, piece (50g)	●	27.6	0.5	248	2	14.5
Carrot cake, slice (75g)	●	39.6	0.6	283	2.6	12
Chocolate cake, slice (75g)	●	42.3	1	268	4.3	10.5
Chocolate mini roll, each (50g)	●	26.6	0.5	210	2.7	10.5
Chocolate sandwich sponge, slice (50g)	●	23.4	0.6	189	2.9	9.5
Date and walnut loaf, slice (75g)	●	32.4	1.1	287	4.7	15.4

TIP: The nutritional values of cakes will vary from one manufacturer to the next, so check the packaging if you need to be precise.

Food type	GI	Carb (g)	Fibre (g)	Cal (kcal)	Pro (g)	Fat (g)
Chocolate éclair, each (75g)	●	19.5	0.6	297	4.2	23.2
Fancy cake, iced, each (50g)	●	34.4	–	204	1.9	7.5
Flapjack, oat, each (75g)	●	45.3	2	363	3.4	20.3
Fruit cake, slice (75g):	●					
plain	●	43.4	–	265.5	3.8	9.8
rich	●	44.9	1.1	257	2.9	8.5
rich, iced	●	47	1.3	267	3	8.3
wholemeal	●	39.6	1.8	272	4.5	12
Ginger cake, slice (75g)	●	45.1	0.9	291	2.6	11.2
Greek pastries (sweet),	●					
each (50g)		20	–	161	2.4	8.5
Lemon cake, slice (75g)	●	41.6	0.8	289	3.4	13.5
Marble cake, slice (75g)	●	41.5	0.9	278	3.9	10..5
Madeira cake, slice (75g)	●	43.8	0.7	295	4	12.8
Mince pie, each (50g)	●	27.9	0.7	184	1.75	7
Sponge cake, slice (50g):						
plain	●	26.2	0.4	234	3.2	13.6
fat-free	●	26.5	0.4	147	5	3
jam-filled	●	32.1	0.9	151	2.1	2.5
with butter icing	●	26.2	0.3	245	2.3	15.5
Swiss roll, original, slice (50g)	●	30.2	0.6	146	2.6	1.6
Trifle sponge, each (50g)	●	33.5	0.5	162	2.6	16

TIP: If the sea of red traffic lights on these pages doesn't put you off craving cake, look at the high fat and calorie counts per slice.

BAKING PRODUCTS

Several of the GI diets include recipes for bran muffins, oatmeal cookies and other baked treats. They keep the GI count down by keeping the fibre count high. Wholemeal flour is best for slow sugar release and adding plenty of dried fruits, nuts and seeds will help as well. Rick Gallop suggests using sugar substitutes, but this is up to you. Some prefer using soya flour, which is medium GI (see page 197) and you could even use ground nuts instead of flour to bring the GI right down.

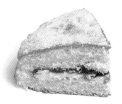

TIP: Wherever possible use stoneground or wholemeal flour for home baking. You may need to add a little more liquid than the recipe advises but the release of glucose into the blood will be much slower than from refined flours.

Food type	GI	Carb (g)	Fibre (g)	Cal (kcal)	Pro (g)	Fat (g)
Baking Agents						
Baking powder, 10g (3tsp)	●	3.8	–	16.3	0.5	–
Cornflour, 25g	●	20.9	–	88	0.2	0.2
Flour, 100g:						
rye, whole	◐	75.9	11.7	335	8.2	20
wheat, brown	●	68.5	6.4	323	12.6	1.8
wheat, white, breadmaking	●	75.3	3.1	341	11.5	1.4
wheat, white, plain	●	77.7	3.1	341	9.4	1.3
wheat, white, self-raising	●	75.6	3.1	330	8.9	1.2
wheat, wholemeal	◐	63.9	9	310	12.7	2.2
Ground rice, 100g	●	86.8	0.5	361	6.5	1
Pastry, 50g:						
filo, uncooked	●	31	1	156	4.5	1.5
flaky, cooked	●	23	0.7	280	2.8	20.3
puff, uncooked	●	15	0.8	210	2.5	15.5
shortcrust, cooked	●	27.1	1.1	260	3.3	16.2
shortcrust, mix	●	30.4	1.1	234	3.7	11.6
wholemeal, cooked	●	22.3	3.1	250	4.5	16.1
Sugar, caster, 50g	●	50	–	200	–	–
Yeast, bakers'						
compressed, 25g	◐	0.3	–	13	2.9	0.1
dried, 15g	◐	0.5	–	25	5.3	0.2

TIP: Make a crumble topping using half flour and half rolled oats or barley flakes.

Food type	GI	Carb (g)	Fibre (g)	Cal (kcal)	Pro (g)	Fat (g)
Fats						
Butter, 25g		0.2	–	186	0.2	21
Cooking fat, 25g		–	–	225	–	25
Lard, 1tbsp		–	–	134	–	14.8
Margarine, hard (over 80% animal/vegetable fat), 25g		0.2	–	180	0.1	20
Margarine, soft (over 80% polyunsaturated fat), 25g		0.05	–	187	–	20.7
Suet, shredded, 1 tbsp	●	1.8	0.1	124	–	13
Mixes						
Batter mix, 100g	●	77.2	3.7	338	9.3	1.2
Cheesecake mix, 100g:						
strawberry	●	31.5	–	258	3	12
toffee	●	37.5	–	342	3.2	19.3
Crumble mix, 100g	●	67.6	1.5	422	5.5	16.3
Egg custard mix, no bake, 100g	●	13.5	–	109	3.5	4.5
Madeira cake mix, 100g	●	56	–	339	4.9	12.4
Pancake mix, 100g	●	65.9	2.3	322	13.4	2.5
Victoria sponge mix, 100g	●	52	–	367	6	15

TIP: Remember that most bakery products supply 'empty calories' without nutritional value – and you'll feel hungry an hour or so after eating them when your blood sugar dips down from its spike.

Food type	GI	Carb (g)	Fibre (g)	Cal (kcal)	Pro (g)	Fat (g)
Sundries						
Almonds, flaked/ground, 25g	●	1.7	0.3	153	5.3	14
Cherries, glacé, 25g	○	16.6	0.2	63	0.1	–
Cherry pie filling, 100g	●	21.5	0.4	82	0.4	–
Currants, dried, 25g	○	17	0.5	67	0.6	0.1
Ginger, glacé, 25g	○	18.5	–	76	–	0.2
Lemon juice, 50ml	●	0.8	–	1.8	–	–
Marzipan, 50g	●	33.8	1	202	2.7	7.2
Mincemeat (sweet), 50g	●	31	0.7	137	0.3	2.1
Mixed peel, 25g	○	14.8	–	57.8	–	0.2
Raisins, seedless, 25g	○	17.3	0.5	68	0.5	0.5
Royal icing, 50g	●	49	–	195	0.7	–
Sultanas, 25g	○	17.3	0.5	69	0.7	0.5

TIP: A handful of nuts and raisins makes a good between-meals snack. Eat one at a time for the slowest 'burn'.

BEANS, PULSES AND CEREALS

Beans and pulses are a valuable source of protein, fibre, calcium, potassium, magnesium, iron and B vitamins and the good news is that most are low-GI as well. Adding beans to soups, salads and casseroles will slow down the digestion of the meal. If you buy canned beans and pulses, drain and rinse them before use. Dried beans are cheaper but they take time to soak and then to cook.

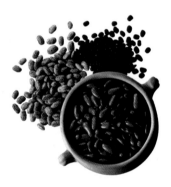

TIP: Make your own baked beans with cannellini beans and fresh tomato sauce, to avoid the high sugar content of tinned baked beans.

Food type	GI	Carb (g)	Fibre (g)	Cal (kcal)	Pro (g)	Fat (g)
Beans and Pulses						
Aduki beans, 115g	●	26	6.3	140	10.6	0.3
Baked beans, small can (200g):						
in tomato sauce	●	30.6	13.8	168	10.4	1.2
tomato sauce, no added sugar	●	17.2	7.4	112	9.4	0.4
Baked beans with pork						
sausages, small can (200g)	●	22.4	5.2	178	11	5
Baked beans with						
vegetable sausages,						
small can (200g)	●	20.4	5.8	192	11.6	7.2
Blackeyed beans, 115g	●	23	4	133	10	0.8
Borlotti beans, half can (100g)	●	20.5	5.5	121	8.7	0.5
Broad beans, small can (200g)	⬤	17	8.4	128	13.4	0.6
Butter beans:						
small can (200g)	●	26	9.2	154	11.8	1
dried, boiled (115g)	●	21	5.9	118	8.1	0.7
Cannellini beans,						
small can (200g)	●	27	12	168	13.6	0.6
Chick peas:						
small can (200g)	●	32.2	8.2	230	14.4	5.4
dried, boiled (115g)	●	20.8	4.9	138	9.6	2.4

TIP: Serve haricot or flageolet beans with roast lamb instead of potatoes. Roast the lamb with garlic and rosemary and mix a little of the flavoured meat juice into the cooked beans before serving.

Food type	GI	Carb (g)	Fibre (g)	Cal (kcal)	Pro (g)	Fat (g)
Chilli beans, small can (200g)	●	27.6	7.4	158	9.6	1
Flageolet beans, half can (100g)	●	22.4	2.4	132	9.0	0.7
Haricot beans, 115g						
dried, boiled	●	19.6	7	109	7.5	0.6
Hummus, 2 tbsp	●	6.2	1.6	53	1.5	2.6
Lentils, 115g:						
green/brown, boiled	●	19.3	4.3	120	10	0.8
red, split, boiled	●	20	2.2	114	8.7	0.5
Marrow fat peas:						
small can (200g)	●	24.6	9.8	154	11.8	1
quick-soak, 115g	●	47.9	16	331	28.9	2.7
Mung beans, 115g						
boiled	●	17.4	3.4	104	9	0.5
Pinto beans:						
boiled, 115g	●	27.3	_	157	10.1	0.8
refried, 2 tbsp	●	4.6	_	32	1.9	0.3
Red kidney beans:						
small can (200g)	●	35.6	17	200	13.8	1.2
boiled, 115g	●	19.8	10.3	118	9.6	0.6
Soya beans, 115g						
dried, boiled	●	5.8	7	161	16	8.3

TIP: Dried mung beans are a good storecupboard standby. Sprinkle them on salads or stews. They're a great source of protein and some experts claim they are useful for cleansing the liver.

Food type	GI	Carb (g)	Fibre (g)	Cal (kcal)	Pro (g)	Fat (g)
Split peas, 115g, *boiled*	●	25.9	3.1	144	9.5	1
Tofu (soya bean curd), 2 tbsp:						
steamed	●	0.9	–	94	10.4	5.4
fried	●	2.6	–	337	30	22.8
Cereals						
Barley, pearl, 100g	●	83.6	7.3	360	7.9	1.7
Bran, 100g:						
wheat, dry	●	26.8	39.6	206	14.1	5.5
soya, cooked	●	15	55	169	16	5
Bulgur wheat, dry, 100g	●	75	1.8	354	11	1.5
Couscous, dry, 100g	●	72.5	2	355	23.5	1.9
Cracked wheat, 100g	●	75	1.8	354	11	1.5
Polenta, ready-made, 100g	●	15.7	–	71.9	1.6	0.3
Wheatgerm, 100g	●	44.7	15.6	302	26.7	9.2
Fresh beans & peas:						
see Vegetables						
For more soya products:						
see Vegetarian						

TIP: Pearl barley makes a good base for a 'risotto' instead of the traditional arborio rice. It takes a little longer to cook but has a delicious nutty flavour and an interesting chewy texture.

BISCUITS, CRACKERS AND CRISPBREADS

Sweet biscuits have no place on any kind of diet, because of their high sugar, fat and calorie content. Savoury crackers and crispbreads are much better; check the fibre content on the label and choose the highest, but beware of high salt content. Biscuits often contain trans fats – hydrogenated or partially hydrogenated fats – so read the label and make sure you avoid them. Most manufacturers provide a 'per biscuit' nutritional breakdown which should help you to distinguish the worst offenders.

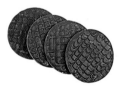

TIP: Coarse oatcakes make a satisfying snack on their own or could be spread with nut butter or hummus. Alternatively, make your own biscuits using oats and dried fruits – many of the GI diets have recipes.

Food type	GI	Carb (g)	Fibre (g)	Cal (kcal)	Pro (g)	Fat (g)
Sweet Biscuits						
Bourbon creams, each	●	7	–	47	–	1.9
Caramel wafers, each	●	6.8	–	45	0.5	2
Chocolate chip cookies, each	●	6.6	0.1	43	0.5	1.6
Chocolate cream wafers, each	●	31.6	–	26	0.3	1.4
Chocolate fingers, each:						
milk & plain chocolate	●	6.4	0.1	53	0.7	2.7
white chocolate	●	6.3	0.1	53	0.7	2.8
Shortcake cream sandwich						
fruit	●	9.2	0.3	75	0.9	3.8
milk chocolate	●	9.4	0.3	77	0.9	3.9
mint	●	9.4	0.3	78	0.8	4
orange	●	9.3	0.3	78	0.8	4.1
Custard creams, each	●	7	0.2	51	0.6	2.3
Digestive biscuits, each:	●	10.3	0.7	71	0.9	3.1
uncoated	◗	8.1	0.8	59	0.8	2.5
chocolate (milk & plain)	●	10	0.5	74	1	3.6
Fig rolls each	●	6.8	0.4	35	0.4	0.8
Garibaldi (plain), each	●	6.7	0.3	40	0.6	1.2
Gingernuts, each	●	7.9	0.1	46	0.6	1.5
Gipsy creams, each	●	9.9	0.4	77	0.7	3.9
Jaffa cakes, each	●	7.4	0.1	38	0.4	0.8
Lemon puff, each	●	5.8	0.2	54	0.6	3.1
Nice biscuits, each	●	6.9	0.4	46	0.7	1.7
Oat & raisin biscuits, each	◗	6.3	0.4	47	0.8	2.1

Food type	GI	Carb (g)	Fibre (g)	Cal (kcal)	Pro (g)	Fat (g)
Rich tea biscuits, each	●	7.7	0.2	48	0.7	1.6
Shortbread fingers, each	●	12.8	0.4	100	1.2	5.2
Shortcake biscuits, each	●	6.7	0.2	48	0.6	2
Stem ginger cookies, diet, each	●	6.5	0.1	40	0.5	1.3
Viennese whirls, each	●	7.7	0.2	75	0.6	4.6
Wafer biscuits, cream-filled, each	●	4.6	n/a	37	0.3	2
Crackers and Crispbreads						
Bran crackers, 4	●	12.6	0.4	91	1.9	3.6
Cheese crackers , 4	●	8.3	0.4	81	1.5	4.7
Cornish wafers, each	●	5.4	0.2	53	0.8	0.2
Crackerbread, each:						
original	●	7.9	0.3	38	1	0.3
cheese-flavoured	●	7.5	0.3	38	1.3	0.3
high-fibre	●	6	1.7	32	1.2	0.3
Crackers, salted, 5:						
cheese	●	8.3	0.3	74	1.6	3.8
original	●	8.3	0.3	76	1	4.3
Cream crackers, each	●	5.3	0.3	34	0.8	1
Matzo crackers, each	●	7.7	0.6	34	1	–
Oatcakes, each:						
cheese	●	5.5	0.6	47	1.4	2.5

TIP: The higher the fibre count of a cracker or crispbread, the lower the glycaemic load should be.

Food type	GI	Carb (g)	Fibre (g)	Cal (kcal)	Pro (g)	Fat (g)
Oatcakes, *contd*:						
fine	●	6.6	0.9	44	1	1.9
organic	●	6.5	0.8	43	1	0.8
rough	●	6.5	0.6	43	1	0.6
traditional	●	6.4	0.8	44	1.2	1.8
Rye crispbread, each:						
dark rye	●	5.6	1.7	27	0.9	0.2
multigrain	●	6.4	1.8	37	1.3	0.7
original	●	5.7	1.6	27	0.8	0.2
sesame	●	3.9	1.4	31	0.9	0.6
Water biscuits, 3:						
high bake	●	7.6	0.3	41	1	0.3
regular (table)	●	8.2	0.3	44	1	0.3
Wholemeal crackers, 4	●	10.8	0.6	62	1.6	1.7

See also Snacks and dips

TIP: Dried fruits in a biscuit will lower the glycaemic load. See page 84 for the low-down on muesli bars.

BREAKFAST CEREALS AND CEREAL BARS

Breakfast is an essential GI diet meal. Without a good intake of slow-release fuels at the beginning of the day, the tendency to snack on sugary foods mid morning will be difficult to overcome. Choose breakfast cereals containing oats or bran and without added sugar. It is easy to make your own basic muesli and to add fresh berries, dried fruits, nuts and seeds. Porridge is a staple low GI breakfast and can be varied with added ingredients. Choose cereal bars with a high fibre content and avoid the chocolate coating.

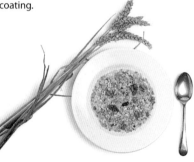

TIP: Always read the ingredient and nutrition labels carefully on breakfast cereals and avoid those with high sugar levels. Look for the flash 'no added sugar'.

Food type	GI	Carb (g)	Fibre (g)	Cal (kcal)	Pro (g)	Fat (g)
Breakfast Cereals						
Bran flakes, 30g	●	20.1	4.5	99	3	0.6
Cheerios, 40g:	●	30.4	2.5	148	3.2	1.5
honey-nut	●	31.3	2.3	149	2.8	1.5
Cornflakes, 30g:	●	25.3	0.7	111	2.1	0.2
Crunchy nut	●	24.9	0.8	117	1.8	1
Sugar coated	●	26.1	0.6	111	1.4	0.1
Chocolate sugar coated	●	24.6	0.9	117	1.4	1.4
Fruit 'n' Fibre, 30g	●	21	2.7	105	2.4	1.5
Grape Nuts, 40g	●	29	3.4	138	4.2	0.8
High Fibre Bran, 40g	◐	18.4	10.8	112	5.6	1.8
Low fat flakes, 30g:	◐	22.2	0.9	111	4.8	0.3
with red berries	◐	22.5	1.2	111	4.2	0.3
Malted Wheats, 30g	●	23.5	1.7	108	3.2	1.5
Multi-grain cereal, 30g	◐	24.6	1.2	111	2.1	0.6
Oat Bran Flakes, 30g	◐	20.1	0.6	99	3	0.6
Oat Krunchies, 30g	◐	18.9	3.3	108	3.1	2.1
Puffed Rice, 30g:	●	26.1	0.3	114	1.8	0.3
chocolate	●	25.5	0.6	114	1.4	0.8
sugar coated	●	27	0.3	114	1.2	0.2
Puffed Wheat, 30g	●	18.7	1.7	98	4.6	0.4

TIP: When choosing cereals, look for the ones with the highest fibre count – at least 5g per serving, if possible. These will provide the steadiest release of fuel through the morning.

Breakfast Cereals and Cereal Bars

Food type	GI	Carb (g)	Fibre (g)	Cal (kcal)	Pro (g)	Fat (g)
Shredded wheat bisks, 30g:	●	19.8	3.4	99	3.4	0.6
bitesize	●	20.3	3.5	100	3.4	0.7
sugar coated	●	21.6	2.7	105	3	0.6
fruit-filled	●	20.7	2.7	96	2.7	0.6
honey nut	●	20.6	3	114	3.3	2
Sultana Bran, 30g	●	20.4	3.6	96	2.4	0.6
Wheat bisks , 30g	●	20.3	3.2	102	3.4	0.8
Hot Cereals						
Instant Porridge						
baked apple	●	71	5.5	374	8	6
berry burst	●	71	5.5	374	8	6
golden syrup	●	72	5	376	7.5	6
Oatbran, 100g	●	49.7	15.2	345	14.8	9.7
Oatmeal, medium or fine, 100g	●	60.4	8.5	359	11	8.1
Oats, 100g:						
instant	●	60.4	8.5	359	11	8.1
jumbo	●	60.4	8.5	359	11	8.1
organic	●	60.4	8.5	359	11	8.1
rolled	●	62	7	368	11	8

TIP: Avoid quick-cook porridge oats, which are stripped of their husks. Traditional oats take longer to cook but are high-fibre and full of vitamins and minerals. Porridge can lower your cholesterol levels and help to prevent heart disease.

Food type	GI	Carb (g)	Fibre (g)	Cal (kcal)	Pro (g)	Fat (g)
Porridge (cooked), 100g:						
made with water	●	9	0.8	49	1.5	1
made with whole milk	●	13.7	0.8	116	4.8	5.1
Muesli						
Crunchy Oat Cereal, 50g:						
maple & pecan	●	30.0	3.2	224	5	9.3
raisin & almond	●	33	2.5	205	4.2	6.
sultana & apple	●	29.6	6.2	189	3.8	6.1
Muesli, 50g:	●	33	3.8	182	5	3.4
apricot	●	29.6	2.8	142	3.8	1.8
deluxe	●	28.1	5.8	172	5.4	5
high fibre	●	35.4	3	158	5.2	3
natural	●	31.5	4.3	173	4.8	3.1
organic	●	31.2	4.6	190	5	5.1
swiss-style	●	36.5	3.2	182	4.9	3
swiss-style, organic	●	31.4	3.7	180	4.8	3.8
with no added sugar	●	33.5	3.9	183	5.2	3.9

TIP: To make your own low-GI muesli, mix oat flakes, rye flakes, millet, pumpkin and sunflower seeds, hazelnuts and dried or chopped fresh fruit. Serve with low-fat cows' or soya milk, or unsweetened natural yoghurt.

Food type	GI	Carb (g)	Fibre (g)	Cal (kcal)	Pro (g)	Fat (g)
Cereal Bars						
Apple & blackberry, 30g	●	21.9	0.9	126	1.7	3.5
Banana, 30g	●	27.6	2	152	2.3	2
Cornflakes & milk bar, 30g	○	19.8	0.6	132	2.7	4.8
Fruit & Nut Break, 30g	○	23.2	3	137	2.6	3.8
Fruit and oats crisp, 30g:						
Apricot	○	21.3	2.1	122	1.7	3.3
Raisin & Hazelnut	○	20.4	1.3	142	2.1	5.8
Low fat flakes & milk bar, 30g	○	20.7	0.4	135	2.1	4.8
Muesli bar, 30g	○	30.6	2	178	2.7	5
Multi-grain bar, 30g:						
Apple	○	20.4	0.9	10.8	1.0	2.7
Cappuccino	○	19.8	0.7	111	1.4	3
Cherry	○	20.4	0.9	108	1.2	2.7
Chocolate	○	19.8	1.0	114	1.4	3.3
Orange	○	20.4	1.2	11.1	1.5	2.7
Strawberry	○	20.4	0.9	10.8	1.2	2.7
Oat and wheat bar, 30g:						
Chocolate chip	●	17.8	n/a	159	2.4	8.7
Roasted nut	○	19.3	n/a	147	1.9	7

TIP: Many cereal bars on the market are simply sugar-coated cereals formed into a bar, sometimes with extra sweeteners and chocolate toppings. Muesli bars with dried fruit, nuts and seeds can be a healthier option, but they should still be an occasional treat on a GI diet.

Food type	GI	Carb (g)	Fibre (g)	Cal (kcal)	Pro (g)	Fat (g)
Puffed rice & milk bar, 30g	●	20.7	0.4	135	2.1	4.8
Strawberry & yoghurt, 30g	●	22.2	0.9	125	1.7	3.3
Sugar coated flakes & milk bar, 30g	●	20.7	1.4	132	2.4	4.5

TIP: To make your own muesli bars, mix together 150g melted butter, 3 tbsps honey, 75g soft brown sugar, 350g porridge oats, 50g raisins and ½ tsp cinnamon. Mash two bananas and stir in to the mixture. Spoon into an oiled 23 x 33cm tin and bake at 180°C or gas mark 4 for 20–25 minutes. Cut into fingers and cool in the baking tin. Store in an airtight container.

CONDIMENTS, SAUCES AND GRAVY

Many ready-made sauces, pickles and chutneys are high in sugar and flour and should be used sparingly on a GI – or any – diet. Home-made condiments and sauces are usually best, especially for marinades, stocks and low-carb sauces. In most cases the need for sugar and flour can be overcome by the use of other more GI-friendly ingredients. Oriental flavours like the Thai lemongrass, ginger, garlic and soy and the Indian spices mixed with natural yoghurt are low GI, as is the Italian combo of tomato, garlic and herbs.

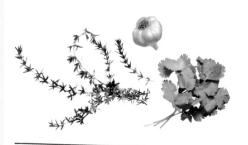

TIP: Don't thicken gravy with flour or gravy powder. Instead, serve the natural meat juices, which could be bulked out with vegetable cooking water, as a thin gravy, called 'jus' in the best restaurants. A spoonful of wine or sherry will make all the difference.

Food type	GI	Carb (g)	Fibre (g)	Cal (kcal)	Pro (g)	Fat (g)
Table Sauces						
Apple sauce, 1 tbsp	●	3.8	0.2	16	–	–
Barbecue sauce, 1 tbsp	●	4.3	–	18	0.2	–
Beetroot in redcurrant jelly 1 tbsp	●	6.6	0.1	25	0.1	–
Brown fruity sauce, 1 tbsp	●	3.6	0.2	17	0.1	–
Brown sauce, 1 tbsp	●	3.8	0.1	15	0.2	–
Burger sauce, 1 tbsp	●	1.6	–	89	0.3	9
Chilli sauce, 1 tsp	●	1.6	–	7	0.1	–
Cranberry jelly, 1 tbsp	●	10	–	40	–	–
Cranberry sauce, 1 tbsp	●	6.8	0.1	27	–	–
Garlic sauce, 1 tsp	●	0.9	–	17	0.1	1.5
Ginger sauce, 1 tsp	●	1.4	–	6	–	–
Horseradish, creamed, 2 tsp	●	2	0.2	18	0.2	1
Horseradish relish, 2 tsp	●	1	0.3	11	0.2	0.6
Horseradish sauce, 2 tsp	●	1.8	0.3	15	0.3	0.8
Mint jelly, 1 tbsp	●	9.9	–	40	–	–
Mint sauce, 1 tbsp	●	2	–	9	0.3	–
Mushroom ketchup, 1 tbsp	●	0.8	–	4	0.1	–
Redcurrant jelly, 1 tbsp	●	9.8	–	39	–	–
Soy sauce, 2 tsp	●	0.8	–	4	0.8	–

TIP: Mint sauce is easy and inexpensive to make. Chop a handful of mint leaves and cover with 1 or 2 tablespoons of white wine vinegar. Add a little sugar or sweetener, to taste.

Food type	GI	Carb (g)	Fibre (g)	Cal (kcal)	Pro (g)	Fat (g)
Tabasco, 1 tsp	–	–	–	–	–	–
Tartare sauce, 1 tbsp	●	1.2	–	77	0.2	8
Tomato ketchup, 1 tbsp	●	3.7	0.1	16	0.1	–
Wild rowan jelly, 2 tsp	●	6.7	–	27	–	–
Worcestershire sauce, 1 tsp	●	1.1	–	4	0.2	–
Mustards						
Dijon mustard, 1 tsp	●	0.3	0.2	6	0.3	0.5
English mustard, 1 tsp	●	1	0.1	9	0.4	0.5
French mustard, 1 tsp	●	0.7	–	7	0.4	0.2
Honey mustard, 1 tsp	●	1.2	0.3	9	0.3	0.2
Horseradish mustard, 1 tsp	●	1.2	0.2	8	0.3	0.2
Peppercorn mustard, 1 tsp	●	0.8	0.3	7	0.4	0.3
Wholegrain mustard, 1tsp:	●	0.8	0.2	7	0.4	0.2
hot, 1 tsp	●	0.6	0.4	7	0.4	0.2
Pickles and Chutneys						
Apple chutney, 1 tbsp	●	7.8	0.2	30	0.1	–
Barbecue relish, 1 tbsp	●	4.4	0.2	20	0.3	0.1
Chunky fruit chutney, 1 tbsp:	●	5.1	0.2	21	0.1	–
small chunk	●	–	0.2	21	0.1	–

TIP: Traditional roast accompaniments: serve unsweetened apple purée or grainy mustard with pork, freshly made mint sauce with lamb and grated horseradish in low-fat crème fraiche with beef.

Food type	GI	Carb (g)	Fibre (g)	Cal (kcal)	Pro (g)	Fat (g)
Chunky fruit chutney, *contd*:						
spicy	●	5.1	0.2	21	0.1	–
Lime pickle, 1 tbsp	●	2.2	0.4	23	0.3	1.4
Mango chutney, 1 tbsp	●	9.2	0.1	42	–	0.5
Mango with ginger chutney 1 tbsp	●	6.9	0.1	28	0.1	–
Mediterranean chutney, 1 tbsp	●	3.9	0.2	17.9	0.3	0.1
Mustard pickle, mild, 1 tbsp	●	4	0.1	19	0.4	0.2
Piccalilli, 1 tbsp	●	3	0.1	13	0.8	–
Ploughman's pickle, 1 tbsp	●	4	0.1	17	0.1	–
Sandwich pickle, tangy, 1 tbsp	●	4.8	0.2	20	0.1	–
Sauerkraut, 2 tbsp	●	0.4	0.6	3	0.4	–
Spiced fruit chutney, 1 tbsp	●	5.2	0.1	21	0.1	–
Spreadable chutney, 1 tbsp	●	7.5	0.2	30	0.1	–
Sweet chilli dipping sauce, 1 tbsp	●	7.8	0.1	33	0.1	–
Sweet pickle, 1 tbsp	●	5.2	0.2	20	0.1	–
Tomato chutney, 1 tbsp	●	6.1	0.2	24	0.2	–
Tomato pickle, tangy, 1 tbsp	●	3.5	0.3	25	0.3	–
Tomato with red pepper chutney, 1 tbsp	●	5.7	0.2	25	0.3	

TIP: To make your own ketchup, blend some finely chopped tomatoes, red pepper, red onion and garlic with cider vinegar and a little molasses (to taste). Store in the refrigerator.

Food type	GI	Carb (g)	Fibre (g)	Cal (kcal)	Pro (g)	Fat (g)
Salad Dressings						
Balsamic dressing, 2 tbsp	●	2.2	–	92	0.1	9.1
Blue cheese dressing, 2 tbsp	●	2.6	–	137	0.6	13.9
Blue cheese-flavoured low-fat dressing, 2 tbsp	●	1.7	–	18	0.5	1
Creamy Caesar dressing, 2 tbsp	●	2.4	–	101	0.9	9.6
Caesar-style low-fat dressing, 2 tbsp	●	1.7	–	18	0.5	1
Creamy low-fat salad dressing, 2 tbsp	●	4.3	–	36	0.3	1.9
French dressing, 2 tbsp	●	1.4	–	139	–	14.8
Italian dressing, 2 tbsp	●	1.6	0.2	35	–	3
fat free	●	1.9	0.2	9	–	–
Mayonnaise, 1 tbsp	●	0.2	–	109	0.2	11.8
light, reduced calorie, 1 tbsp	●	1	–	45	0.1	5
Salad cream, 1 tbsp	●	2.5	–	52	0.2	4.7
light, 1 tbsp	●	1.9	–	35	0.2	3
Seafood sauce, 1 tbsp	●	14.8	0.1	80	0.2	8.1
Thousand Island, 1 tbsp	●	2.9	–	54	0.1	4.6
fat free, 1 tbsp	●	2.9	0.4	12	0.1	–
Vinaigrette, 2 tbsp	●	1.4	–	139	–	14.8

TIP: Mix your own salad dressing either in a jar or in the bottom of the salad bowl. Use twice as much oil as vinegar or lemon juice and add fresh chopped herbs, crushed garlic and mustard as flavourings.

Food type	GI	Carb (g)	Fibre (g)	Cal (kcal)	Pro (g)	Fat (g)
Vinegars						
Balsamic vinegar, 1 tbsp	●	3.2	–	15	–	–
Cider vinegar, 1 tbsp	●	0.2	0.1	3	–	–
Red wine vinegar, 1 tbsp	●	0.1	–	4	–	–
Sherry vinegar, 1 tbsp	●	0.3	–	4	–	–
White wine vinegar, 1 tbsp	●	0.1	–	3	–	–
Cooking Sauces						
Bread sauce, 100ml:						
made with semi-skimmed milk	●	11.1	0.6	128	4.2	1
made with whole milk	●	10.9	0.6	150	4.1	10.3
Cheese sauce, 100ml:						
made with semi-skimmed milk	●	8.8	0.2	181	8.2	12.8
made with whole milk	●	8.7	0.2	198	8.1	14.8
Curry sauce, canned, 100ml	●	7.1	–	78	1.5	5
Onion sauce, 100ml:						
made with semi-skimmed milk	●	8.4	0.4	86	2.9	5
made with whole milk	●	8.3	0.4	99	2.8	6.5
Pesto:						
fresh, homemade 100ml	●	6	1.4	45	2.2	1.3
green pesto, jar, 100ml	●	3.5	1.4	427	4.7	43.8

TIP: Shop-bought cook-in sauces can be high-GI. When you read the label, watch out for the quantity of sugars, and note how near the top of the ingredients list sugar appears.

Food type	GI	Carb (g)	Fibre (g)	Cal (kcal)	Pro (g)	Fat (g)
Pesto contd:						
red pesto, jar, 100ml	●	3.1	0.4	358	4.1	36.6
Tomato & basil, fresh, 100ml	●	8.8	1.3	51	1.8	0.9
White sauce, 100ml:						
made with semi-skimmed milk	●	10.7	0.2	130	4.4	8
made with whole milk	●	10.6	0.2	151	4.2	10.3
For more pasta sauces, see under: Pasta and Pizza						
Stock Cubes						
Beef, each	●	4.2	0.2	29	1.9	0.5
Chicken, each	●	4	0.2	27	1.2	0.4
Fish, each	●	1.8	0.1	36	2.1	2.2
Garlic herb & spice, each	●	5.3	0.4	33	1.5	0.6
Ham , each	●	2.7	–	34	1.3	2
Lamb, each	●	4.8	0.2	32	1.7	0.6
Rice saffron, each	●	1.4	0.4	32	1.6	2.2
Pork, each	●	1.9	–	37	1.3	2.7
Vegetable, each	●	4.6	0.2	28	1.2	0.5
Yeast extract, each	●	2.8	–	27	2.8	0.6

TIP: Stir grated cucumber into low-fat natural yoghurt and serve as an Indian-style accompaniment to meats. Alternatively, make a tomato salsa with tomatoes, red onion, basil and balsamic vinegar.

Food type	GI	Carb (g)	Fibre (g)	Cal (kcal)	Pro (g)	Fat (g)
Gravy Granules						
Gravy powder, 5g	●	2.99	0.06	12	0.1	0.01
Gravy instant granules, 5g	●	2.0	–	23	0.2	1.6
Swiss Vegetable						
Bouillon powder, 4g	●	1.1	–	11	0.4	0.5
Vegetable gravy granules, 5g	●	2.98	0.05	16	0.4	0.25

TIP: To make your own vegetable stock, slice an onion, 2 leeks, a fennel bulb and 2 carrots. Add some fresh parsley, coriander seeds, bay leaves and thyme, cover with water and simmer for 45 minutes, then strain.

DAIRY

Most dairy foods don't have a GI rating because they don't contain any carbohydrate and therefore don't affect blood sugar levels. The exceptions are milk and yoghurt, which contain a sugar called lactose. To lose weight and have a healthy heart, you should opt for low-fat versions of dairy products. Most cheeses, butters and creams are high in saturated fats, which could raise your cholesterol levels and clog up your arteries.

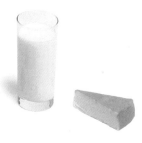

TIP: Whole milk has a lower GI value than skimmed milk, but the authors of all the GI diets still recommend that you opt for skimmed or low-fat dairy products to protect your heart. Unsweetened soya milk is an even healthier option.

Food type	GI	Carb (g)	Fibre (g)	Cal (kcal)	Pro (g)	Fat (g)
Milk and Cream						
Buttermilk, 250ml	●	13.8	–	100	10.8	0.3
Cream:						
extra thick, 2 tbsp	●	1.1	–	88	0.7	9
fresh, clotted, 2 tbsp	●	0.7	–	176	0.5	19
fresh, double, 2 tbsp	●	0.5	–	149	0.5	16.1
fresh, single, 2 tbsp	●	0.7	–	58	1	5.7
fresh, soured, 2 tbsp	●	0.9	–	62	1.1	6.0
fresh, whipping, 2 tbsp	●	0.8	–	114	0.6	12
sterilised, canned, 2 tbsp	●	1.1	–	76	0.6	7.2
UHT, aerosol spray, 2 tbsp	●	2.2	–	86	0.7	7.2
UHT, double, vegetarian, 2 tbsp	●	1.2	0.1	105	0.7	10.8
UHT, single, vegetarian, 2 tbsp	●	1.4	0.06	44	0.9	3.9
Crème fraiche:						
full fat, 2 tbsp	●	19	–	113	0.5	0.7
half fat, 2 tbsp	●	4.5	–	49	0.8	1.3
Milk, fresh:						
cows', whole, 250ml	●	11.3	–	165	82.5	9.8
cows', semi-skimmed, 250ml	●	11.8	–	115	8.5	4.25
cows', skimmed, 250ml	●	11	–	80	8.5	0.5
cows', Channel Island, 250ml	●	12.8	–	195	9	12

TIP: Cheeses only register on the GI scale if they have added ingredients like fruit, nuts or herbs. For the sake of your health, opt for low-fat, low-calorie cheeses like feta, edam and mozzarella.

Food type	GI	Carb (g)	Fibre (g)	Cal (kcal)	Pro (g)	Fat (g)
Milk, *contd:*						
goats', pasteurised, 250ml	●	11	–	155	7.8	9.3
sheep's, 250ml	●	9.3	–	150	7.8	11
Milk, evaporated:						
original, 100ml	●	54.3	–	330	8.3	9.1
light, 100ml	●	10.3	–	107	7.8	4.1
Milk, dried, skimmed, 250ml	●	11.0	–	870	90.3	1.5
Milk, condensed:						
whole milk, sweetened, 100ml	●	55.5	–	333	8.5	10.1
skimmed milk, sweetened, 100ml	●	60	–	267	10	0.2
Soya milk:						
unsweetened, 250ml	●	1.3	0.5	65	6	4
sweetened, 250ml	●	6.3	–	108	7.8	6
Rice drink:						
calcium enriched, 250ml	●	25	–	125	0.3	2.8
vanilla, organic, 250ml	●	25	–	123	0.3	2.5
Yoghurt and Fromage Frais						
Diet yoghurts, 125g:						
banana	●	10.9	n/a	66	5.5	0.1
cherry	●	9.9	n/a	62	5.5	0.1
vanilla	●	10.4	n/a	66	5.7	0.1

TIP: Fruit yoghurts can be high in sugar and the diet ones are usually sweetened artificially. Add fresh fruits to plain yoghurt instead.

Food type	GI	Carb (g)	Fibre (g)	Cal (kcal)	Pro (g)	Fat (g)
Fromage frais, 1 pot (50g):						
fruit	●	6.9	–	62	2.6	2.8
plain	●	2.8	–	56	3.4	3.5
virtually fat free, fruit	●	2.8	0.2	25	3.2	0.1
virtually fat free, plain	●	2.3	–	25	3.8	0.05
Fruit corner, 125g:						
blueberry	●	18.9	n/a	140	4.6	4.9
strawberry	●	21.4	n/a	148	4.6	4.9
Greek-style, cows, fruit, 1 pot (125g)	●	14	–	171	6	10.5
Greek-style, cows, plain, 1 pot (125g)	●	6	–	166	7.1	12.7
Greek-style, sheep, 1 pot (125g)	●	6.25	–	115	6	7.5
Low fat, fruit, 1 pot (125g)	●	17.1	0.25	98	5.2	1.4
Low fat, plain, 1 pot (125g)	●	9.25	–	70	6	1.25
Natural bio yoghurt, 125g	●	7	–	68	5.5	1.9
Orange fat-free bio yoghurt each	●	11.3	0.1	61	5.4	0.2
Raspberry drinking yoghurt, per bottle	●	12.5	0.1	78	2.9	1.8
Soya, fruit, 1 pot (125g)	●	16.1	0.4	91	2.6	2.25
Virtually fat free, fruit, 1 pot (125g)	●	8.75	–	59	6	0.25

TIP: Probiotic yoghurts and spreads can help to lower cholesterol and improve digestive functioning.

Food type	GI	Carb (g)	Fibre (g)	Cal (kcal)	Pro (g)	Fat (g)
Virtually fat free, plain, 1 pot (125g)	●	10.2	–	67.5	6.8	0.25
Yoghurt drink, 125ml:						
natural	●	8.6	n/a	84	6.9	2.4
peach	●	16.2	n/a	94	3.2	1.8
Whole milk, fruit, 1 pot (125g)	●	22.1	–	136	5	3.75
Whole milk, plain, 1 pot (125g)	●	9.8	–	99	7.1	3.75
Butter and Margarine						
Butter:						
lightly salted, 15g		–	–	108	–	12
spreadable, 15g		0.1	–	112	–	12
salted, 15g		0.1	–	112	0.1	12.3
Margarine, hard						
animal & vegetable fat,						
over 80% fat, 15g		0.1	–	108	–	12
Margarine, soft						
polyunsaturated, over 80%						
fat, 15g		0.03	–	112	–	12.4
Spreads						
Olive oil spread, 15g		0.1	–	80	–	8.8

TIP: Don't avoid dairy products altogether: they are an important source of calcium, which helps to prevent osteoporosis.

Food type	GI	Carb (g)	Fibre (g)	Cal (kcal)	Pro (g)	Fat (g)
Olive oil spread, *contd:*						
very low fat (20-25%)		0.4	–	39	0.9	3.8
Polyunsaturated spread:						
buttery, 15g		0.07	–	95	0.06	10.5
light, 15g		0.5	0.1	54	–	5.7
low salt, 15g		–	–	95	–	10.5
sunflower spread, 15g		–	–	95	–	10.5
Pro-biotic, 15g		–	–	86	–	9.6
light		–	–	48	–	5.4
Cheeses						
Bel Paese, individual, 25g		–	–	77	5.8	6
Bavarian smoked, 25g		0.1	–	69	4.3	5.8
Brie, 25g		–	–	86	5.1	7.3
Caerphilly, 25g		–	–	92	5.8	8
Cambozola, 25g		0.1	–	108	3.4	10.4
Camembert, 25g		–	–	72	5.4	5.7
Cheddar:						
English, 25g		–	–	104	6.4	8.8
vegetarian, 25g		–	–	98	1.4	8
Cheddar-type, half fat, 25g		–	–	68	8.2	4

TIP: Use monounsaturated oils like olive or rapeseed in place of butter. You can dip bread into a saucer of oil, or even use oil for baking, where it will give lighter results than butter or margarine.

Food type	GI	Carb (g)	Fibre (g)	Cal (kcal)	Pro (g)	Fat (g)
Cheshire, 25g		–	–	95	6	7.9
Cottage cheese:						
plain, 100g	●	3.1	–	101	12.6	4.3
reduced fat, 100g	●	3.3	–	79	13.3	1.5
with additions, 100g	●	2.6	–	95	12.8	3.8
Cream cheese, full fat, 25g		–	–	110	0.8	12
ail & fines herbs, 25g		0.5	–	104	1.8	10.5
au naturel, 25g		0.5	–	106	1.8	10.8
au poivre, 25g		0.5	–	104	1.8	10.5
Danish Blue, 25g		–	–	86	5.1	7.2
Dolcelatte, 25g		0.2	–	99	4.3	9
Double Gloucester, 25g		–	–	101	6.1	8.5
Edam, 25g		–	–	85	6.7	6.5
Emmenthal, 25g		0.1	–	103	6.3	8.6
Feta, 25g		0.4	–	63	3.9	5
Goats' milk soft cheese, 25g		0.3	–	80	5.3	6.5
Gorgonzola, 25g		–	–	78	4.8	9
Gouda, 25g		–	–	94	6.2	7.7
Grana Padano, 25g		–	–	96	8.3	7
Gruyère, 25g		–	–	99	6.8	8
Jarlsberg, 25g		–	–	90	6.8	7
Lancashire, 25g		–	–	95	5.9	8

TIP: Use a potato peeler to cut extra thin slices of cheese. These look attractive on top of a salad.

Food type	GI	Carb (g)	Fibre (g)	Cal (kcal)	Pro (g)	Fat (g)
Mascarpone, 25g		0.8	–	105	0.9	11.1
Mature cheese, reduced fat, 25g		–	–	77	6.8	5.5
Medium-fat soft cheese, 25g		0.9	–	49.8	2.5	4
Mild cheese, reduced fat, 25g		–	–	77	6.8	5.5
Mozzarella, 25g		–	–	64	4.7	5
Parmesan, fresh, 25g		0.2	–	103.8	9	7.4
Quark, 25g		1	–	15	2.8	–
Red Leicester, 25g		–	–	100	6	8.4
Ricotta, 25g		0.5	–	34	2.3	2.5
Roquefort, 25g		–	–	89	5.8	7.3
Sage Derby, 25g		0.7	–	104	6.1	8.5
Shropshire blue, 25g		–	–	102	5.6	8.9
Soft cheese:						
full fat, 25g		0.8	–	63	1.5	6
light medium fat, 25g		0.9	–	48	1.9	4
light with chives, 25g		0.9	–	46	1.9	3.8
light with tomato & basil, 25g	●	1.1	0.1	45	1.9	3.5
Stilton:						
blue, 25g		–	–	103	5.9	8.8
white, 25g		–	–	90	5	7.8
white, with apricots, 25g	●	2.6	–	88	4.2	6.8
Wensleydale, 25g		–	–	94	5.7	7.9

TIP: Use wholemeal breadcrumbs and grated cheese as an 'au gratin' topping for vegetables and casseroles.

Food type	GI	Carb (g)	Fibre (g)	Cal (kcal)	Pro (g)	Fat (g)
Wensleydale, *contd*:						
with cranberries, 25g	●	2.4	–	92	5.3	6.8
Cheese Spreads and Processed Cheese						
Cheese spread:						
original, 25g	●	0.5	–	60	3.3	5
cheese & chive, 25g	●	0.3	–	59	3.2	5
cheese & shrimp, 25g	●	0.5	–	60	3.3	5
cheese & ham, 25g	●	0.4	–	59	3.2	5
cheese & garlic, 25g	●	1	–	62	3.9	5
light, 25g	●	1.7	–	43	4	5
Cheese slices:	●					
singles, 25g	●	1.9	–	65	3.4	3.7
singles light, 25g	●	1.5	–	51	5	2.8
Cheese triangles, 25g	●	1.8	–	56	2.5	4.4
Processed cheese, plain, 25g	●	1.3	–	74	2	5
Strip cheese, 25g	●	0.5	–	90	6.1	6.9

TIP: The following dairy products get the 'green light' on Rick Gallop's *GI Diet*: buttermilk, fat-free cheese, fat-free cottage cheese, low-fat/no-sugar ice cream, skimmed milk, fat-free sour cream and no-fat/no-sugar yoghurt.

Food type	GI	Carb (g)	Fibre (g)	Cal (kcal)	Pro (g)	Fat (g)
See also: Jams, Marmalades and Spreads For ice cream: *see under Desserts and Puddings*						

TIP: Make a fondue with 250g grated gruyère or emmenthal cheese, 1 crushed garlic clove, 150ml dry white wine, and 2 level tsps cornflour. Blend together over a low heat. Add a tbsp of dried cherries and dip in strips of raw vegetables. Makes a sociable meal. (Non dieters can eat crusty bread with it.)

DESSERTS AND PUDDINGS

These are two words which shouldn't be in the GI dieter's vocabulary because you won't find any green traffic lights in this section. Every so often the temptation might prove too strong or it might be rude to decline a dessert if you are eating at a friend's house. In this case, take a very small portion or, if possible, choose unsweetened fresh fruit salad or fresh fruit as an alternative.

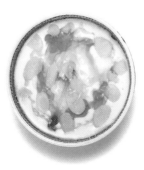

TIP: Rather than a traditional pudding, a better GI dessert is a platter of seasonal fruit, which will not need added sugar. Tropical fruits like kiwi, lychees and passion fruit are all naturally sweet.

Food type	GI	Carb (g)	Fibre (g)	Cal (kcal)	Pro (g)	Fat (g)
Puddings						
Bread pudding, 100g	●	48	1.2	289	5.9	9.5
Christmas pudding, 100g	●	56.3	1.7	329	3	11.8
Creamed rice, 100g	●	15.2	–	90	3.1	1.9
Meringue, 100g	●	95.4	–	379	5.3	–
Pavlova, with raspberries, 100g	●	45	–	297	2.5	11.9
Profiteroles, 100g	●	18.5	0.4	358	6.2	29.2
Rice pudding, 100g:	●	19.6	0.1	130	4.1	4.3
with sultanas & nutmeg	●	16.6	0.1	105	3.2	2.9
Sago pudding, 100g:						
made with semi-skimmed milk	●	20.1	0.1	93	4	0.2
made with whole milk	●	19.6	0.1	130	4.1	4.3
Semolina pudding, 100g:						
made with semi-skimmed milk	●	20.1	0.1	93	4	0.2
made with whole milk	●	19.6	0.1	130	4.1	4.3
Sponge pudding:						
with chocolate sauce, 100g	●	48.2	1.4	285	2.7	9.1
lemon, 100g	●	50.1	0.6	306	2.7	10.6
treacle, 100g	●	49.2	0.6	278	2.3	8
Spotted Dick, 100g	●	51.2	2.3	357	5.7	15
Tapioca pudding, 100g:						
made with semi-skimmed milk	●	20.1	0.1	93	4	0.2

TIP: Sliced apples and pears will not go brown if they are sprinkled with lemon juice.

Food type	GI	Carb (g)	Fibre (g)	Cal (kcal)	Pro (g)	Fat (g)
Tapioca pudding, 100g, *contd:*						
made with whole milk	●	19.6	0.1	130	4.1	4.3
Trifle, 100g	●	22.3	0.5	160	3.6	6.3
Trifle with fresh cream, 100g	●	19.5	0.5	166	2.4	9.2
Sweet Pies and Flans						
Apple & blackcurrant pies, each	●	52.7	1.5	331	3.4	13
Apple pie, 100g	●	35.3	0.9	235	2.8	9.6
Bakewell tart, 100g	●	56.7	0.9	397	3.8	17
cherry bakewell	●	58.5	1.2	412	3.9	18
Cheesecake, 100g:	●	33	0.9	242	5.7	10.6
raspberry	●	31.9	0.6	299	4.7	17.2
Custard tart, 100g	●	32.4	1.2	277	6.3	15
Dutch apple tart, 100g	●	34.4	0.6	237	3.2	9.9
Fruit pie, individual:	●	56.7	–	369	4.3	16
pastry top & bottom, 100g	●	34	1.8	260	3	13
wholemeal one crust, 100g	●	26.6	2.7	183	2.6	8.1
Jam tart, 100g	●	63.4	–	368	3.3	13
Lemon meringue pie, 100g	●	45.9	0.7	319	4.5	14
Mince pies, 100g	●	56.8	1.5	372	3.8	14
luxury, 100g	●	55.7	1.5	387	3.7	14
Treacle tart, 100g	●	60.4	1.1	368	3.7	1.1

TIP: Cut thin slices of peeled pineapple and grill both sides briefly under a hot grill. Serve with a sprig of mint.

Food type	GI	Carb (g)	Fibre (g)	Cal (kcal)	Pro (g)	Fat (g)
Chilled and Frozen Desserts						
Crème brulée, 100g	●	23.5	0.2	251	1.3	17
Crème caramel, 100g	●	20.6	–	109	3	2.2
Chocolate nut sundae, 100g	●	26.2	0.2	243	2.6	14.9
Ice cream, 100g:						
Cornish	●	11.3	n/a	92	19	4.4
chocolate	●	20.6	n/a	187	3.5	10.6
Neapolitan	●	20.1	n/a	173	3.6	9.3
peach melba	●	13.2	n/a	94	1.7	3.8
raspberry ripple	●	24.3	n/a	192	3.2	9.8
strawberry	●	10.5	n/a	84	1.7	3.8
tiramisu	●	15.2	n/a	112	2.1	4.6
vanilla	●	11.4	n/a	90	1.5	4.5
Ice cream bar, chocolate-covered, 100g	●	21.8	–	311	5	23.3
Ice cream dessert, frozen, 100g	●	21	–	251	3.5	17.6
Instant dessert powder, 100g:						
made up with whole milk	●	14.8	0.2	111	3.1	6.3
Jelly, 100g, made with water	●	15.1	–	61	1.2	–
Mousse, 100g:						
chocolate	●	19.9	–	139	4	2.1
fruit	●	18	–	137	4.5	5.7

TIP: Make a fruit fool with fresh fruit purée mixed with Greek yoghurt instead of cream.

Food type	GI	Carb (g)	Fibre (g)	Cal (kcal)	Pro (g)	Fat (g)
Sorbet, 100g:						
fruit	●	24.8	–	97	0.2	0.3
lemon	●	34.2	–	131	0.9	–
Tiramisu, 100g	●	31.2	0.3	337	3.5	22.2
Vanilla soya dessert, each	◐	16.4	1.3	101	3.8	2.3
For yoghurt, *see under Dairy*						
Toppings and Sauces						
Brandy flavour sauce mix, 50ml	●	38.2	–	208	3.0	4.7
Brandy sauce, ready to serve,						
50ml	◐	8.2	–	48	1.4	0.8
Chocolate custard mix, 50ml:						
chocolate flavour	●	39.3	0.1	208	3.0	4.4
low fat	●	39.3	0.1	202	2.2	4.1
Custard, 50ml:						
made with skimmed milk	◐	8.4	–	40	1.9	0.05
made with whole milk	◐	8.3	–	59	1.8	2.2
canned or carton	◐	7.8	–	51	1.4	1.5
Devon custard, canned, 50ml	◐	8.2	0.05	52	1.4	1.5
Artificial cream topping, 50ml	●	16.2	0.25	345	3.4	29.3
sugar-free	●	15.2	0.25	348	3.6	30.2

TIP: Stuff some apples with sultanas or raisins and chopped nuts, but no sugar. Rub the skins with oil and cut a slit round the middle before baking in a hot oven for 20 minutes.

Food type	GI	Carb (g)	Fibre (g)	Cal (kcal)	Pro (g)	Fat (g)
Maple syrup, organic, 1 tsp	●	3.4	–	13	–	–
Rum sauce (Bird's), 50ml	●	7.8	–	46	1.4	0.8
White sauce, sweet, 50ml						
made with semi-skimmed milk	●	9.3	0.1	76	2	3.7
made with whole milk	●	9.2	0.1	86	2	4.8

TIP: Peel some pears and stew gently in a mixture of equal quantities of red wine and water. A piece of cinnamon bark adds flavour. When they are soft, serve with low-fat yoghurt or ice cream.

DRINKS

Most diets advise that you drink at least eight full glasses of still water every day, and it should be your drink of choice on a GI diet. Fruit juices, squashes and cordials can all produce a blood sugar high, because they don't have the fibre to slow the absorption of fructose that would be found in the equivalent fruit. Tea and coffee are stimulants but are carb-free if drunk without sugar and milk. Most GI diets recommend that you avoid alcohol during the weight-loss phase and only allow yourself one glass of wine or one beer a day when you have reached your target weight.

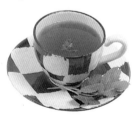

TIP: Caffeine in tea, coffee and cola drinks is a stimulant and may cause a rise in insulin which will upset the digestion of starches and sugars, so limit the number of cups to three or four per day.

Food type	GI	Carb (g)	Fibre (g)	Cal (kcal)	Pro (g)	Fat (g)
Alcoholic						
Advocaat, 25ml	◐	7.1	–	68	1.2	5.3
Beer, bitter, 500ml:	●					
canned	●	11.5	–	160	1.5	–
draught	●	11.5	–	160	1.5	–
keg	●	11.5	–	155	1.5	–
Beer, mild draught, 500ml	●	8.0	–	25	1.0	–
Brandy, 25ml		–	–	56	–	–
Brown ale, bottled, 500ml	●	15	–	140	1.5	–
Cider, 500ml:						
dry	◐	13	–	180	–	–
sweet	●	21.5	–	210	–	–
vintage	●	36.5	–	505	–	–
Cognac, 25ml		–	–	88	–	–
Gin, 25ml		–	–	56	–	–
Lager, bottled, 500ml	●	7.5	–	145	1.0	–
Pale ale, bottled, 500ml	●	10	–	160	–	–
Port, 25ml	◐	3	–	39	0.1	–
Rum, 25ml		–	–	56	–	–
Sherry, 25ml						
dry	●	0.4	–	29	0.1	–
medium	●	0.8	–	30	–	–

TIP: 'Lite' beers are lower in calories than ordinary beer but they also have a higher sugar content and therefore a higher GI value.

Food type	GI	Carb (g)	Fibre (g)	Cal (kcal)	Pro (g)	Fat (g)
Sherry, contd						
sweet	●	2	–	4	0.1	–
Stout, 500ml:						
bottled	●	21	–	185	1.5	–
extra	●	10.5	–	195	1.5	–
Strong ale, 500ml	●	30.5	–	360	3.5	–
Vermouth, 50ml:						
dry	●	2.75	–	59	0.05	–
sweet	●	8.0	–	76	–	–
bianco	–	–	–	72	–	–
extra dry	–	–	–	48	–	–
rosso	–	–	–	70	–	–
Vodka, 25ml	–	–	–	56	–	–
Whisky, 25ml	–	–	–	56	–	–
Wine, per small glass (125ml):						
red	●	0.4	–	85	0.2	–
rosé	●	3.1	–	89	0.1	–
white, dry	●	0.8	–	82	0.1	–
white, medium	●	4.2	–	94	0.1	–
white, sparkling	●	7.4	–	95	0.2	–
white, sweet	●	7.4	–	117	0.2	–

TIP: Although some alcoholic drinks don't have a GI value, it doesn't mean you can drink unlimited quantities because they are full of empty calories, as well as challenging your liver.

Food type	GI	Carb (g)	Fibre (g)	Cal (kcal)	Pro (g)	Fat (g)
Liqueurs						
Cherry, 25ml	●	8.2	–	63.8	–	–
Coffee, 25ml	●	n/a	–	66	–	–
Coffee cream, 25ml	●	n/a	–	80	–	–
Orange, 25ml	●	n/a	–	85	–	–
Triple sec, 25ml	●	n/a	–	80	–	–
Juices and Cordials						
Apple juice, unsweetened, 250ml	○	24.8	–	95	0.3	0.3
Apple & elderflower juice, 250ml	○	25.5	–	108	1	–
Apple & mango juice, 250ml	○	25.3	–	108	1	–
Barley water, 250ml:						
lemon, original	●	49	–	220	0.8	–
no added sugar	○	27.5	–	28	0.5	–
orange, original	●	52.5	–	223	0.8	–
Blackcurrant & apple juice, 250ml	●	31.3	–	125	–	–
Carrot juice, 250ml	○	14.3	–	60	1.3	0.3
Cranberry juice, 250ml	○	25.2	–	110	–	–

TIP: Standard mixers will lift the GI value of alcoholic drinks sky-high. Gin and tonic, rum and coke, and whisky and ginger are all high-GI and high-calorie options.

Food type	GI	Carb (g)	Fibre (g)	Cal (kcal)	Pro (g)	Fat (g)
Grape juice, unsweetened, 250ml	○	29.3	–	115	0.8	0.3
Grapefruit juice, 250ml	○	22	0.8	90	0.5	–
Lemon squash, low calorie, 250ml	○	1	–	5	0.3	–
Lime juice cordial, undiluted, 25ml	○	6.1	–	26	–	–
Orange & mango fruit juice, 250ml	●	26	–	115	1.5	–
Orange & pineapple fruit juice, 250ml	●	27.5	–	120	1.3	–
Orange juice, unsweetened, 250ml	○	22	0.3	90	1.3	0.3
Orange squash, low calorie, 250ml	○	6	–	25	0.3	–
Pineapple juice, unsweetened, 250ml	○	26.3	0.3	103	0.8	0.3
Tomato juice, 250ml:	○	7.5	1.5	35	2	–
cocktail (Britvic), 250ml	○	8	–	47	2.3	0.3

TIP: Black and green teas have high levels of antioxidants that are good for your heart and may help prevent some cancers. A number of health benefits are claimed for herbal teas: mint soothes the digestive system, dandelion cleanses the liver, lemon balm can lift your mood, chamomile is relaxing and can also relieve headaches.

Food type	GI	Carb (g)	Fibre (g)	Cal (kcal)	Pro (g)	Fat (g)
Fizzy Drinks						
Apple drink, sparkling, 330ml	●	38.3	–	155	–	–
Bitter lemon, 355ml	●	27	–	112	–	–
Cherry Coke, 330ml	●	37	–	148	–	–
Cherryade, 330ml	●	–	–	4	–	–
Cola, 330ml	●	35	–	142	–	–
diet	●	–	–	2	–	–
Cream Soda, 330ml	●	23.8	–	96	–	–
Dandelion & Burdock, 330ml	●	17.8	–	74	–	–
Ginger Ale, American 330ml	●	30.4	–	126	–	–
Ginger Ale, Dry 330ml	●	12.5	–	53	–	–
Ginger beer, 330ml	●	28	–	120	–	–
Irn Bru, 330ml	●	33.3	–	135	–	–
diet, 330ml		–	–	2.3	–	–
Lemon drink, sparkling, 330ml	●	37.3	–	155	–	–
low calorie	●	0.3	–	3	–	–
Lemonade, 330ml	●	18.5	–	69	–	–
low calorie		–	–	3	–	–
Glucose drink, 330ml	●	59.1	–	241	–	–
Orange drink, 330ml	●	22.1	–	95	–	–
low calorie	●	2.3	–	18	–	–

TIP: Sports drinks are the antithesis of what a GI dieter is trying to achieve. They are mainly glucose and formulated to give an instant energy (i.e. blood sugar) high.

Food type	GI	Carb (g)	Fibre (g)	Cal (kcal)	Pro (g)	Fat (g)
Ribena, sparkling, 330ml	●	43.9	–	178	–	–
low calorie	●	0.3	–	7	–	–
Tonic water, 330ml	●	16.8	–	72	–	–
Water, flavoured, 330ml	●	0.7	–	3.3	–	–
Hot and Milky Drinks						
Beef instant drink, per mug	●	9.75	–	452	99	–
Cappuccino, per sachet:						
instant	●	12	–	72	2	1.7
unsweetened	●	9.8	–	77	2.7	3
Chicken instant drink, per mug	●	48.5	5.2	322	24	3.5
Cocoa, per mug						
made with semi-skimmed milk	●	17.5	0.5	142	8.7	4.8
made with whole milk	●	17.0	0.5	190	8.5	10.5
Coffee, black, per mug	●	–	–	–	0.25	–
Coffee creamer, per tsp	●	3.9	–	35	0.1	1.9
virtually fat free, per tsp	●	5	–	25	0.1	0.8
Drinking chocolate, per mug						
made with semi-skimmed milk	●	27	–	178	8.7	4.7
made with whole milk	●	26.5	–	225	8.5	10.2
Espresso, per 100ml	●	10	1.1	104	15.2	0.4

TIP: Bottled and canned fizzy drinks are high in sugar. The diet versions are free of sugar but artificial sweeteners don't have a good press. Best of all is water, which can also act as a hunger depressant.

Food type	GI	Carb (g)	Fibre (g)	Cal (kcal)	Pro (g)	Fat (g)
Herb teas, per mug	●	–	–	–	0.1	–
Ice tea, per mug	●	18	–	75	–	–
Malted milk, per mug						
made with semi-skimmed milk	●	32.5	–	198	9.8	6.7
made with whole milk	●	27.2	–	242	9.5	9.5
Malted milk light,						
made with water, per mug	●	55.8	2.2	305	11	3.5
Strawberry milkshake, 250ml						
made with semi-skimmed milk	●	62.2	–	387	17	8.5
made with whole milk	●	47.2	–	420	17	19.5
Tea, black, per cup		–	–	–	0.1	–

TIP: Watch out for the sugar content in fruit juices. Even the freshly squeezed juices may be high. Much better to eat a piece of fresh fruit and the fibre will slow down the transfer of sugar into the blood.

EGGS

Eggs contain a wealth of nutrients and are a particularly good source of vitamin E. They are also carb free but the egg yolks do contain cholesterol, which is why some nutritionists recommend that you cook with the egg whites only. Choose Omega-3 eggs, which are high in healthy fatty acids, and boil or poach rather than frying.

TIP: Many nutritionists recommend that you eat some protein at breakfast time, because it is a 'brain food' that helps to switch on the neurotransmitters that relay messages to and from your brain.

Food type	GI	Carb (g)	Fibre (g)	Cal (kcal)	Pro (g)	Fat (g)
Eggs, chicken, 1 medium:						
raw, whole		0.6	–	78	6.3	5.3
raw, white only		0.3	–	17	3.5	–
raw, yolk only		0.3	–	59	2.8	5.1
boiled		0.6	–	76	6.3	5.3
fried, in vegetable oil		0.6	–	93	7	7
poached		0.6	–	76	6.3	5.3
Eggs, duck, raw, whole		0.6	–	84	7.3	6
Omelette (2 eggs, 10g butter):						
plain	●	1.2	–	228	12.6	18.6
with 25g cheese	●	1.3	–	475	27.8	39.5
Scrambled (2 eggs with						
15 ml milk, 20g butter)	●	1.9	–	310	13	27.1

TIP: Use fresh, lightly steamed vegetables with a little low-fat cheese as a filling for a nutritious omelette. Cook in a non-stick pan brushed or sprayed with olive oil.

FISH AND SEAFOOD

Oily fish like salmon, herrings, mackerel, sardines and tuna are rich in valuable Omega-3 fatty acids, which protect the arteries and strengthen the immune system. White fish are a valuable protein source with a wide variety of textures and flavours available. Shellfish should be looked on as an occasional treat as prawns, in particular, contain cholesterol.

The only GI prohibition in this section is to avoid fish coated in batter or breadcrumbs or served with flour-based sauces.

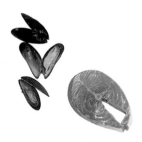

TIP: Make an Italian salad with canned tuna and white haricot and butter beans, jazzed up with a few rings of red onion and a spoonful of chopped parsley. Sprinkle with lemon juice.

Food type	GI	Carb (g)	Fibre (g)	Cal (kcal)	Pro (g)	Fat (g)
Fish and Seafood						
Anchovies, in oil,						
drained, 100g		–	–	280	25.2	19.9
Cockles, boiled, 100g		–	–	48	17.2	2
Cod:						
baked fillets, 100g		–	–	96	21.4	1.2
dried, salted, boiled, 100g		–	–	138	32.5	0.9
in batter, fried, 100g	●	11.7	0.5	247	16.1	15.4
in crumbs, fried, 100g	●	15.2	–	235	12.4	14.3
in parsley sauce, boiled, 100g	●	2.8	–	84	12	2.8
poached fillets, 100g		–	–	94	20.9	1.1
steaks, grilled, 100g		–	–	95	20.8	1.3
Cod roe, hard, fried, 100g	●	3	0.1	202	20.9	11.9
Coley fillets, steamed, 100g		–	–	99	23.3	0.6
Crab						
boiled, 100g		–	–	127	20.1	5.2
canned, 100g		–	–	81	18.1	0.9
dressed, 100g		–	–	105	16.9	14.2
Eels, jellied, 100g		–	–	98	8.4	7.1
Haddock:						
in crumbs, fried, 100g	●	12.6	–	196	14.7	10

TIP: When cooking fish, remember that less is more. Allow a few minutes on each side under a hot grill, or steam in a fish kettle. If you are baking fish in the oven, wrap it in foil so it doesn't dry out.

Food type	GI	Carb (g)	Fibre (g)	Cal (kcal)	Pro (g)	Fat (g)
Haddock, *contd*:						
smoked, steamed, 100g		–	–	101	23.3	0.9
steamed, 100g		–	–	98	22.8	0.8
Halibut, steamed, 100g		–	–	131	23.8	4
Herring:						
fried, 100g	●	1.5	–	234	23.1	15.1
grilled, 100g		–	–	199	20.4	13
Kippers, grilled, 100g		–	–	205	25.5	11.4
Lemon sole:						
steamed, 100g		–	–	91	20.6	0.9
goujons, baked, 100g	●	14.7	–	187	16	14.6
goujons, fried, 100g	●	14.3	–	374	15.5	28.7
Lobster, boiled, 100g		–	–	119	22.1	3.4
Mackerel, fried, 100g		–	–	188	21.5	11.3
Mussels, boiled, 100g		–	–	87	17.2	2
Pilchards,						
canned in tomato sauce, 100g	●	0.7	–	126	18.8	5.4
Plaice						
in batter, fried, 100g	●	12	–	257	15.2	16.8
in crumbs, fried, 100g	●	8.6	–	228	18	13.7
goujons, baked, 100g	●	27.7	–	304	8.8	18.3

TIP: Instead of coating fishcakes or fish fillets with egg and bread-crumbs, coat in rolled oats, medium oatmeal or finely chopped almonds or walnuts.

Food type	GI	Carb (g)	Fibre (g)	Cal (kcal)	Pro (g)	Fat (g)
Plaice, contd:						
goujons, fried, 100g	●	27	–	426	8.5	32.3
steamed, 100g		–	–	93	18.9	1.9
Prawns: shelled, boiled, 100g		–	–	107	22.6	1.8
boiled, weighed in shells, 175g		–	–	72	15	1.2
king prawns, freshwater, 100g		–	–	70	16.8	0.3
North Atlantic, peeled, 100g		–	–	61	15.1	0.1
tiger king, cooked, 100g		–	–	61	13.5	0.6
Roe:						
cod, hard, fried, 100g	●	3	0.1	202	20.9	11.9
herring, soft, fried, 100g	●	4.7	–	244	21.1	15.8
Salmon:						
pink, canned in brine, drained, 100g		–	–	155	20.3	8.2
grilled steak, 100g		–	–	215	24.2	13.1
smoked, 100g		–	–	142	25.4	4.5
steamed, flesh only, 100g		–	–	197	20.1	13
Sardines:						
canned in oil, drained, 100g		–	–	217	23.7	13.6
canned in tomato sauce, 100g	●	0.9	–	177	17.8	11.6
Scampi tails, premium, 100g	●	26	–	230	8.4	10.9

TIP: Avoid creamy and mayonnaise sauces with shellfish. Much better to use freshly squeezed lemon or lime, or a tomato salsa, and serve with a fresh salad.

Food type	GI	Carb (g)	Fibre (g)	Cal (kcal)	Pro (g)	Fat (g)
Shrimps:						
canned, drained, 100g	–	–	94	20.8	1.2	
frozen, without shells, 100g	–	–	73	16.5	0.8	
Skate, fried in butter, 100g	●	4.9	0.2	199	17.9	12.1
Sole: *see* Lemon sole						
Swordfish, grilled, 100g	●	1.4	–	139	17	9.9
Trout:						
brown, steamed, 100g	–	–	135	23.5	4.5	
rainbow, grilled, 100g	–	–	135	21.5	5.4	
Tuna, fresh, grilled, 100g	–	–	215	24.2	13.1	
canned in brine, 100g	–	–	99	23.5	0.6	
canned in oil, 100g	–	–	189	27.1	9	
Whelks, boiled,						
weighed with shells, 100g	–	–	14	2.8	0.3	
Whitebait, fried, 100g	●	5.3	0.2	525	19.5	47.5
Whiting:						
steamed, flesh only, 100g	–	–	92	20.9	0.9	
in crumbs, fried, 100g	●	7	0.3	191	18.1	10.3
Winkles, boiled,						
weighed with shells, 100g	–	–	14	2.9	0.3	

TIP: Ceviche is a delicious raw fish salad with a very low GI value. Cut firm fish like halibut or salmon into cubes and marinade in fresh lime juice for about an hour. Add a sliced half avocado, a few olives and a finely chopped chilli (optional). Serve on shredded lettuce.

Food type	GI	Carb (g)	Fibre (g)	Cal (kcal)	Pro (g)	Fat (g)
Breaded, Battered or in Sauces						
Calamari in batter, 100g	●	15.8	0.7	299	13.7	20.4
Fish cakes, 100g						
fried, each	●	15.1	–	188	9.1	10.5
Fish fingers						
fried in oil, 100g	●	17.2	0.6	233	13.5	12.7
grilled, 100g	●	19.3	0.7	214	15.1	9
oven crispy, 100g	●	15.8	0.4	218	10.4	12.6
Fish steaks in butter sauce, 100g	●	2.9	0.1	93	9.4	4.9
Fish steaks in parsley sauce, 100g	●	2.9	0.1	85	9.4	4.9
Kipper fillets with butter, 100g		–	–	205	15	16
Prawn Cocktail (Lyons), 100g	●	4.5	–	429	5.7	42.9
Seafood sticks, 100g	●	14.1	–	97	10.7	14.1
Shrimps, potted, 100g		–	–	358	16.5	32.4

TIP: Canned sardines or rollmop herrings go well with chopped celery and sliced apple. Grilled mackerel and gooseberry sauce is a classic combination. Or try Antony Worrall Thompson's recipe for a low-GI fish pie.

FRUIT

All fruits naturally contain fructose, which will have an effect on your blood sugar when it is digested. Don't peel fruit unnecessarily, because the fibre in the peel will slow the absorption of the fruit sugar. To minimise the impact, eat fruit after a main course or with some other low- or no-GI value food. Choose organically grown fruits in season and buy unwaxed citrus fruits to avoid the pesticide residues which are one of the downsides of modern growing methods.

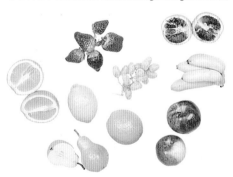

TIP: A study published in the journal of the American College of Nutrition showed that dried figs and prunes are high in antioxidants, which have protective anti-cancer properties.

Food type	GI	Carb (g)	Fibre (g)	Cal (kcal)	Pro (g)	Fat (g)
Apple, 1 medium	●	21	3.8	82	0.2	0.6
Apples, stewed						
with sugar (60g)	●	11.5	0.7	144	0.2	0.06
without sugar (60g)	●	4.9	0.9	19.8	0.2	0.06
Apricots: 1 fresh	●	3.9	0.8	16	0.5	0.1
dried, 8 halves	●	17	2.5	66	1	0.2
canned in juice, 100g	●	8.4	0.9	34	0.5	0.1
canned in syrup, 100g	●	16.1	0.9	63	0.4	0.1
Avocado, half medium	●	8	3.4	160	1.9	16.4
Banana, 1 medium	●	23.2	3.1	95	1.2	0.3
Blackberries:						
fresh, 75g	●	3.8	2.3	19	0.7	0.2
stewed with sugar, 75g	●	10.4	1.8	42	0.5	0.05
stewed without sugar, 75g	●	3.3	1.9	15	0.6	0.05
Blackcurrants:						
fresh, 75g	●	4.9	2.7	21	0.7	–
stewed with sugar, 75g	●	11.2	2.1	44	0.5	–
canned in syrup, 75g	●	13.8	2.7	54	0.5	–
Blueberries, fresh, 75g	●	7.6	1.6	32	0.4	0.2
Cherries, half cup fresh (90g)	●	10.4	0.8	43	0.8	0.09
Cherries, glacé, 25g	●	16.6	0.2	63	0.1	–

TIP: Start breakfast with a citrus fruit salad: mix slices of pink and white grapefuit or pomelo with oranges and mandarins and garnish with mint leaves.

Food type	GI	Carb (g)	Fibre (g)	Cal (kcal)	Pro (g)	Fat (g)
Clementines, 1 medium	●	6.6	0.9	28	0.7	0.1
Coconut:						
creamed, 2 tbsp	●	1.4	n/a	134	1.2	13.7
desiccated, 2 tbsp	●	1.3	2.7	121	1	12.4
milk, 100ml	●	1.6	–	166	1.6	17.0
Cranberries, fresh, 75g	●	4	4.8	17	0.5	–
Damsons:						
fresh, 75g	●	7.2	1.4	28	0.4	–
stewed with sugar (2 tbsp)	●	5.8	0.4	22	0.1	–
Dates, quarter cup (50g)	●	15.6	0.9	62	0.8	0.05
Figs:						
1 fresh	●	9.6	1.7	37	0.4	0.2
dried, ready to eat, 50g	●	24.3	3.5	104	1.6	0.75
canned in syrup, 100g	●	14	–	59	0.5	–
Fruit cocktail, 100g						
canned in juice	●	14.8	1	57	0.4	–
canned in syrup	●	20.1	1	77	0.4	1
Gooseberries:						
fresh, 75g	●	9.7	1.8	40	0.5	0.2
stewed with sugar (2 tbsp)	●	5.5	0.6	22	0.1	–
Grapefruit, half, fresh	●	7.8	1.5	34	0.9	0.1

TIP: Bananas are not low-GI fruits but they should not be cut from your diet long term as they contain valuable nutrients. Their conversion to blood sugars can be slowed down if eaten with a glass of water.

Food type	GI	Carb (g)	Fibre (g)	Cal (kcal)	Pro (g)	Fat (g)
Grapes, black/white, seedless,						
fresh, 75g	●	11.6	0.5	45	0.3	0.75
Greengages:						
fresh, 75g	●	6.4	1.2	26	0.4	–
stewed with sugar (2 tbsp)	●	8	0.4	32	0.4	–
Guavas, fresh, 60g	●	3	2.2	16	0.5	0.3
Honeydew melon: see Melon						
Jackfruit, fresh, 75g	●	16	–	66	1.0	0.2
Kiwi fruit, peeled, each	●	10.6	1.9	49	1.1	0.5
Lemon, whole	●	3.2	n/a	19	1	0.3
Lychees, fresh, 75g	●	10.7	0.5	44	0.7	0.07
canned in syrup, 100g	●	17.7	0.5	68	0.4	–
Mandarin oranges, 100g:						
canned in juice	●	7.7	0.3	32	0.7	–
canned in syrup	●	14.4	0.2	52	0.5	–
Mangos, 1 medium	●	16	0.2	66	0.8	0.2
Melon, fresh, medium slice:						
cantaloupe	●	4.8	1.3	22	0.7	0.1
galia	●	6.4	0.5	27	0.6	0.1
honeydew	●	7.5	0.7	32	0.7	0.1
watermelon	●	8.1	0.1	35	0.6	0.3

TIP: Fruit smoothies can be made easily by whizzing together your choice of fruits with plain yoghurt. Blueberries and raspberries are particularly good.

Food type	GI	Carb (g)	Fibre (g)	Cal (kcal)	Pro (g)	Fat (g)
Nectarines, 1 medium	●	13.5	1.8	60	2.1	0.1
Oranges, 1 medium	●	12.8	2.5	56	1.6	0.1
Papaya, half, fresh	●	10	2.5	41	0.6	0.1
Passionfruit, 75g						
fresh (flesh & pips only)	●	4.4	2.5	27	1.9	0.3
Paw-paw, half, fresh	●	10	2.5	41	0.6	0.1
Peach, 1 medium	●	11.4	2.2	50	1.3	0.1
canned in juice, 100g	●	9.7	0.8	39	0.6	–
canned in syrup, 100g	●	14	0.9	55	0.5	–
Pear, 1 medium	●	15	3.3	60	0.4	0.1
canned in juice, 100g	●	8.5	1.4	33	0.3	–
canned in syrup, 100g	●	13.2	1.1	50	0.2	–
Pineapple, fresh, 60g	●	6.0	0.3	25	0.2	0.1
canned in juice, 100g	●	12.2	0.5	47	0.3	–
canned in syrup, 100g	●	16.5	0.7	64	0.5	–
Plums, 1 medium	●	8.8	1.6	36	0.6	0.1
Prunes, canned in juice, 100g	●	19.7	2.4	79	0.7	0.2
canned in syrup, 100g	●	23	2.8	90	0.6	0.2
Prunes, dried: *see under* Snacks						
Raisins: *see under* Snacks						
Raspberries, fresh, 60g	●	2.8	1.5	15	0.8	0.2

TIP: Beware the added sugar in canned fruit. Even if it is canned in fruit juice, there will still be more sugar than in fresh. Much better to choose whatever is in season for the highest vitamin content.

Food type	GI	Carb (g)	Fibre (g)	Cal (kcal)	Pro (g)	Fat (g)
Rhubarb, fresh, raw, 60g	●	`0.5	0.8	4	0.5	0.06
stewed with sugar (2 tbsp)	●	3.4	0.4	0.3	–	
stewed without sugar (2 tbsp)	●	0.2	0.4	0.3	–	
Satsumas, 1 medium	●	12.8	2	1.4	0.1	
Strawberries, 70g	●	4.2	0.8	0.6	0.07	
Tangerines, fresh, one	●	8	1.3	0.9	0.1	
Watermelon, *see under* Melon						

TIP: Many fruits combine well with savoury flavours in a salad or hot dish. Mangoes go well with cooked chicken; apples with pork; berry fruits with low-fat game; and grapes and citrus fruits with fish.

JAMS, MARMALADES AND SPREADS

Most jams, jellies and marmalades contain a high proportion of easily absorbed sugar; if you must have jam, look for the kinds that contain reduced sugar and extra fruit. Jams specially made for diabetics are a good idea. Never choose a spread where sugar is listed at the top of the ingredients list. Nut butters are low-GI and an excellent source of vitamins and minerals but high in calories, so eat sparingly in the weight-loss phase of your diet. The ever-popular yeast extract should be a staple in every store-cupboard because of its high vitamin B content.

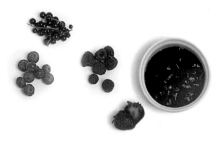

TIP: Nut butters or hummus make good dips served with fresh vegetable strips. If the texture is too firm, mix with a little plain yoghurt. Add a few extra chopped nuts to garnish.

Food type	GI	Carb (g)	Fibre (g)	Cal (kcal)	Pro (g)	Fat (g)
Jams and Marmalades						
Apricot conserve, 1 tsp	●	3.2	–	13	–	–
Apricot fruit spread, 1 tsp:						
diet	●	1.4	–	6	–	–
organic	●	1.8	0.1	7	–	–
Apricot jam, 1 tsp:						
reduced sugar	●	2.7	–	11	–	–
sucrose free	●	3.2	–	–	–	–
Blackcurrant jam, 1 tsp:						
reduced sugar	●	2.7	0.1	11	–	–
sucrose free	●	3.4	–	8.5	–	–
Blueberry & blackberry jam, organic, 1 tsp	●	3	0.1	13	–	–
Grapefruit fruit spread, 1 tsp	●	1.9	0.1	7	–	–
Grapefruit marmalade, 1 tsp	●	3.1	–	12	–	–
Honey, 1 tsp:						
clear	●	3	–	12	–	–
honeycomb	●	3.9	–	14	–	–
set	●	3.9	–	14	–	–
Lemon curd, 1 tsp	●	3	–	14	–	–
Marmalade:						
orange, 1 tsp	●	3.3	–	8	–	–

TIP: If you make your own jams and marmalades you can restrict the amount of sugar you add – but they still won't have low-GI values.

Food type	GI	Carb (g)	Fibre (g)	Cal (kcal)	Pro (g)	Fat (g)
Marmalade, *contd*:						
Dundee, 1 tsp	●	2.7	–	11	–	–
organic, 1 tsp	●	3.2	–	13	–	–
thick-cut, 1 tsp	●	3.5	–	13	–	–
Morello cherry fruit spread						
organic, 1 tsp	●	1.8	0.5	7	–	–
Pineapple & ginger fruit						
spread, 1 tsp	●	1.9	0.1	7	–	–
Raspberry conserve, 1 tsp	●	3.2	–	13	–	–
Raspberry fruit spread, 1 tsp:						
diet	●	1.4	–	6	–	–
organic	●	7.5	–	7	–	–
Raspberry jam, 1 tsp:	●	3.5	0.1	13	–	–
organic	●	3.2	–	13	–	–
reduced sugar	●	2.7	0.1	11	–	–
sucrose free	●	3.2	–	8	–	–
Rhubarb & ginger jam,						
reduced sugar, 1 tsp	●	2.7	–	11	–	–
Seville orange fruit spread, 1 tsp						
reduced sugar	●	1.4	–	6	–	–
organic	●	1.8	0.1	7	–	–

TIP: Yeast extract on toast is a way of life for most British children and rightly so, as the extract is rich in B vitamins. Use it also as a flavouring in soups and casseroles.

Food type	GI	Carb (g)	Fibre (g)	Cal (kcal)	Pro (g)	Fat (g)
Strawberry fruit spread, 1 tsp	●	1.4	–	6	–	–
organic	●	1.8	0.1	7	–	–
Strawberry jam, 1 tsp:						
classic	●	3.2	–	13	–	–
reduced sugar	●	2.7	–	11	–	–
sucrose free	●	3.2	–	8	–	–
Wild blackberry jelly,						
reduced sugar, 1 tsp	●	2.7	0.1	11	–	–
Wild blueberry fruit spread,						
organic, 1 tsp	●	1.8	0.2	7	–	–
Nut Butters						
Almond butter, 1 tsp	●	0.3	–	31	1.3	2.8
Cashew butter, 1 tsp	●	0.9	–	31	1	2.6
Chocolate nut spread, 1 tsp	●	3	–	28	0.3	1.7
Hazelnut butter, 1 tsp	●	0.2	–	34	0.8	3.3
Peanut butter, 1 tsp:						
crunchy	●	0.7	0.3	30	1.4	2.4
smooth	●	0.7	0.4	29	1.4	2.4
organic	●	0.6	0.4	30	1.6	2.4
stripy chocolate	●	1.7	0.2	31	0.7	2.3
Tahini paste, 1 tsp	●	–	0.4	30	0.9	2.9

TIP: Spread tahini on oatcakes, dip crudités into it, or use it to make your own hummus with chickpeas, lemon, garlic and olive oil.

Food type	GI	Carb (g)	Fibre (g)	Cal (kcal)	Pro (g)	Fat (g)
Savoury Spreads and Pastes						
Beef spread, 1 tsp	●	0.1	–	9	0.8	0.6
Cheese spread, 1 tsp:	●	0.2	–	13	0.6	1.1
reduced fat	●	0.4	–	9	0.8	0.5
very low fat	●	0.4	–	7	0.8	0.3
See also under: Dairy						
Chicken spread, 1 tsp	●	0.1	–	8	0.8	0.5
Crab spread, 1 tsp	●	0.3	–	7	0.7	0.3
Fish paste, 1 tsp	●	0.2	–	8	0.8	0.5
Guacamole, 1 tsp:						
reduced fat	●	0.2	0.2	7	0.1	0.6
Hummus, 1 tsp	●	0.6	0.1	9	0.4	0.6
Liver pâté, 1 tsp:	●	0.1	–	16	0.6	1.4
low-fat	●	0.1	–	9.5	0.9	0.6
Meat paste, 1 tsp	●	0.2	–	4	0.8	0.6
Mushroom pâté, 1 tsp	●	0.4	–	12	0.4	0.9
Salmon spread, 1 tsp	●	0.2	–	9	0.7	0.5
Sandwich spread, 1 tsp	●	1.3	–	11	0.1	0.6

TIP: Still not sure about the healthiest spreads to use? Dr Gillian McKeith's *You Are What You Eat Cookbook* has loads of delicious recipe suggestions. Try her Asparagus Spread, Almond Pâté, Sweet Carrot Butter, Sesame Squash Spread or Black Olive Tapenade. It doesn't take long to re-educate your palate to enjoy savoury flavours on toast or crackers rather than sweet.

Food type	GI	Carb (g)	Fibre (g)	Cal (kcal)	Pro (g)	Fat (g)
Sandwich spread, *contd*:	●					
cucumber, 1 tsp	●	0.9	–	9.3	0.1	0.6
Taramasalata, 1 tsp	●	0.4	0.1	26	0.1	2.7
Toast toppers, 1 tsp:	●					
chicken & mushroom	●	0.3	0.01	2.8	0.2	0.07
ham & cheese	●	0.4	–	4.8	0.4	0.2
Tzatziki, 1tsp	●	0.2	–	6.3	0.2	0.5
Yeast extract, half tsp	●	0.7	0.1	12	22	–

TIP: Meat and fish pâtés or low-fat cream cheese on unbuttered oatcakes make a quick nutritious lunch when served with a crunchy mixed salad.

MEAT AND POULTRY

Fresh and frozen meat and poultry do not contain carbohydrates so have no glycaemic count unless they have been processed. Items such as sausages, burgers and black puddings have a 'filler' added and so do have a GI value. Hormones and antibiotics are commonly used in rearing animals so it is wise to buy organic meat or to know the animals' provenance. Watch out for high saturated fat content. Where fat is visible, it can be trimmed away or skimmed off after cooking. Continental sausages and salamis are particularly high. Skinless poultry and game are low.

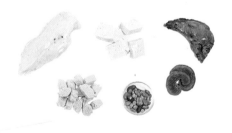

TIP: Chicken and turkey mince have less fat than beef or lamb mince and can be used for home-made burgers or in pasta sauces. Even healthier is soya mince (see page 198).

Food type	GI	Carb (g)	Fibre (g)	Cal (kcal)	Pro (g)	Fat (g)
Cooked Meats						
Bacon, 3 rashers, back (50g):						
dry fried	–	–	–	148	12.1	11
grilled	–	–	–	144	11.6	10.8
microwaved	–	–	–	154	12.1	11.7
Bacon, 3 rashers, middle (50g),						
grilled	–	–	–	154	12.4	11.6
Bacon, 3 rashers, streaky (50g):						
fried	–	–	–	168	11.9	13.3
grilled	–	–	–	169	11.9	13.5
Beef, 100g:						
roast rib	–	–	–	300	29.1	20.4
mince, stewed	–	–	–	209	21.8	13.5
rump steak, lean, grilled	–	–	–	177	31	5.9
rump steak, lean, fried	–	–	–	183	30.9	6.6
sausages, see under Sausages						
silverside, lean only, boiled	–	–	–	184	30.4	6.9
stewing steak, stewed	–	–	–	223	30.9	11
topside, lean only, roasted	–	–	–	202	36.2	6.3
topside, lean & fat, roasted	–	–	–	244	32.8	12.5
Beef grillsteaks, grilled,						
100g	0.5		–	305	22.1	23.9

TIP: Opt for lean back bacon or turkey bacon rather than streaky or other cuts, and trim off all visible fat before grilling.

Food type	GI	Carb (g)	Fibre (g)	Cal (kcal)	Pro (g)	Fat (g)
Burgers, each:						
beefburgers (100g) fried		0.1	–	329	28.5	23.9
beefburgers (100g) grilled		0.1	–	326	26.5	24.4
quarter-pounder (120g)	●	4	0.2	220	17.5	12.7
chicken burger	●	9.6	0.2	150	7.8	8.7
vegetable burger	●	21	1.7	179	2.3	9.5
vegetable quarter-pounder	●	23	1.8	190	4.3	9.1
Black pudding, 2 slices, fried	●	29	0.4	519	18	37.6
Chicken, 100g:						
breast, grilled		–	–	148	32	2.2
breast in crumbs, fried	●	14.8	0.7	242	18	12.7
breast, stir fried		–	–	161	29.7	4.6
1 drumstick, roast		–	–	185	25.8	9.1
1 leg quarter, roast (175g)		–	–	413	45.1	15.9
light & dark meat, roasted		–	–	177	27.3	7.5
light meat, roasted		–	–	153	30.2	3.6
Duck, 100g:						
crispy, Chinese style		0.3	–	331	27.9	24.2
meat only, roasted		–	–	195	25.3	10.4
meat, fat & skin, roasted		–	–	423	20	38.1

TIP: Marinade meats before barbecuing so that they stay moist. Try yoghurt with Indian spices for a masala effect or lemongrass, ginger, lime juice and soy sauce for a Thai flavour. Mix the marinade and put in a plastic bag with the meat, turning so it gets coated evenly.

Food type	GI	Carb (g)	Fibre (g)	Cal (kcal)	Pro (g)	Fat (g)
Gammon, joint, boiled, 100g		–	–	204	23.3	12.3
Gammon, rashers, grilled, 100g		–	–	199	27.5	9.9
Goose, roasted, 100g		–	–	301	27.5	21.2
Haggis, boiled, 100g	●	19.2	–	310	10.7	21.7
Kidney, lamb, fried, 100g		–	–	188	23.7	10.3
Lamb, 100g:						
breast, lean only, roasted		–	–	273	26.7	18.5
breast, lean & fat, roasted		–	–	359	22.4	29.9
cutlets, lean only, grilled		–	–	238	28.5	13.8
cutlets, lean & fat, grilled		–	–	367	24.5	29.9
loin chops, lean only, grilled		–	–	213	29.2	10.7
loin chops, lean & fat, grilled		–	–	305	26.5	22.1
leg, lean only, roasted		–	–	203	29.7	9.4
leg, lean & fat, roasted		–	–	240	28.1	14.2
mince, stewed		–	–	208	24.4	12.3
stewed		–	–	240	26.6	14.8
shoulder, lean only, roasted		–	–	218	27.2	12.1
shoulder, lean & fat, roasted		–	–	298	24.7	22.1
Liver, calf, fried, 100g		–	–	176	22.3	9.6
Liver, chicken, fried, 100g		–	–	169	22.1	8.9

TIP: Lamb neck fillet is easily trimmed of fat and is a good base for kebabs. Cut it into cubes and thread onto skewers along with small onions, cherry tomatoes, chunks of courgette and peppers. In summer, cook it on the barbecue.

Food type	GI	Carb (g)	Fibre (g)	Cal (kcal)	Pro (g)	Fat (g)
Liver, lamb, fried, 100g		–	–	237	30.1	12.9
Oxtail, stewed, 100g		–	–	243	30.5	13.4
Pheasant, roasted, 100g		–	–	220	27.9	12
Pork, 100g:						
belly rashers, grilled		–	–	320	27.4	23.4
loin chops, lean, grilled		–	–	184	31.6	6.4
leg, lean only, roasted		–	–	182	33	5.5
leg, lean & fat, roasted		–	–	215	30.9	10.2
steaks		–	–	162	18	10
Pork sausages: see Sausages						
Rabbit, meat only,						
stewed, 100g		–	–	114	21.2	3.2
Sausages:						
beef sausages (2), grilled	●	14.7	0.8	313	15	21.9
Cumberland sausages (2)	●	3.6	0.4	218	14.2	16.0
Frankfurters (2)	●	2.3	–	377	13.5	34.9
Lincolnshire sausages (2)	●	9.8	1.6	345	14	27.3
pork sausages (2), fried	●	11	0.8	347	15.6	26.9
Saveloy, 100g	●	10.8	0.8	296	13.8	22.3
Tongue, fat & skin removed,						
stewed, 100g		–	–	289	18.2	24
Tripe, dressed, 100g		–	–	33	7.1	0.5

TIP: Red meats naturally contain fats so grill rather than adding more fat with frying. Trim any visible fat before eating.

Food type	GI	Carb (g)	Fibre (g)	Cal (kcal)	Pro (g)	Fat (g)
Turkey, 100g:						
breast fillet, grilled		–	–	155	35	1.7
dark meat, roasted		–	–	177	29.4	6.6
light meat, roasted		–	–	153	33.7	2
Veal, escalope, fried, 100g	○	4.4	–	195	33.7	6.8
Venison, haunch, meat only,						
roasted, 100g		–	–	165	35.6	2.5
White pudding, 100g	●	36.3	–	450	7	31.8
Cold Meats						
Beef, roasted, 50g						
silverside	○	1.2	–	69	9.6	2.9
topside	○	0.2	–	79	12.7	3
Chicken, roasted breast meat,						
50g		–	–	76	15.1	1.8
Chorizo, 50g	○	2	–	19	11.5	15.5
Corned beef, 50g	○	0.5	–	102	13	5.4
Garlic sausage, 50g	○	2.9	0.3	95	7.7	5.8
Ham & pork, chopped, 50g	○	0.7	0.2	138	7.2	11.8
Ham, 50g:						
canned		–	–	60	9.2	2.6
honey-roast	○	1.4	0.5	68	10	2.2

TIP: Venison is a low-fat meat and is now widely available in supermarkets. Try venison mince to make a chilli with red kidney beans.

Food type	GI	Carb (g)	Fibre (g)	Cal (kcal)	Pro (g)	Fat (g)
Ham, contd:						
mustard	●	0.6	0.4	70	11.3	2.5
on the bone	●	0.4	0.3	68	10.4	7.7
beechwood smoked	●	0.25	–	75	10.3	1.3
Parma	●	0.05	–	60	6.4	3.8
Wiltshire	●	0.75	0.55	100	10	6.4
Yorkshire	●	0.6	–	96	7.7	7.9
Haslet, 50g	●	9.3	0.4	72	6.4	1
Kabanos, 50g	●	0.5	0.25	120	12.2	7.7
Liver pâté, 50g	●	0.8	–	348	12.6	32.7
reduced fat	●	3	–	191	18	12
Liver sausage, 50g	●	3	0.4	113	6.7	8.4
Luncheon meat, canned, 50g	●	1.8	0.1	140	6.5	11.9
Pâté, Brussels, 50g	●	0.5	–	163	6.5	15
Pepperami, hot, 50g	●	1.3	0.6	277	9.5	26
Pork salami sausage, 50g	●	0.9	0.1	268	11	24.5
Polony, 50g	●	7.1	–	141	4.7	10.6
Pork, 50g:						
luncheon meat	●	1.6	–	130	7	10.7
oven-baked	●	0.7	0.4	92	13	0.7
Salami, 50g:						
Danish	●	0.3	0.1	219	10.5	19.6

TIP: Serve grilled sausages with a mixed bean salad or home-made baked beans in tomato sauce to lower the overall GI value of the meal.

Food type	GI	Carb (g)	Fibre (g)	Cal (kcal)	Pro (g)	Fat (g)
Salami, *contd:*						
German	●	0.5	–	198	9.5	17.5
Milano	●	1.5	–	214	11.5	18
Scotch eggs, 100g	●	13.1	–	241	12	16
Tongue, lunch, 50g	●	0.2	–	88	9.7	5.2
Turkey, breast, roasted, 50g	●	0.2	0.4	54	11.5	0.8

TIP: Make an antipasti salad with a selection of cold continental cooked meats, olives, grilled peppers and sun-dried tomatoes. Serve with a green salad and breadsticks rather than hunks of bread.

OILS AND FATS

Oils and fats are carb free and therefore have no GI count but they all contain 9 calories of fat per gram – which can mount up to a lot of extra calories when you're frying food. Opt for the ones with the highest levels of monounsaturated fats – such as olive oil and rapeseed oil – and try to avoid saturated fats like suet, lard, beef dripping and coconut oil. See page 26 for more advice on the healthiest oils to use.

TIP: Buy oils in small quantities as flavours go off after they have been stored for a while. Follow suggestions on the bottle for usage as some oils are not suitable for frying or cooking. Expensive olive and nut oils are better used as a salad dressing.

Food type	GI	Carb (g)	Fibre (g)	Cal (kcal)	Pro (g)	Fat (g)
Coconut oil, 1 tbsp		–	–	135	–	13.8
Cooking fat, 1 tbsp		–	–	135	–	15
Corn oil, 1 tbsp		–	–	135	–	15
Dripping, beef, 1 tbsp		–	–	134	–	15
Ghee:						
butter, 1 tbsp		–	–	135	–	15
palm, 1 tbsp		–	–	135	–	15
Lard, 1 tbsp		–	–	134	–	15
Olive oil, 1 tbsp		–	–	135	–	15
Palm oil, 1 tbsp		–	–	135	–	15
Peanut oil, 1 tbsp		–	–	135	–	15
Rapeseed oil, 1 tbsp		–	–	135	–	15
Safflower oil, 1 tbsp		–	–	135	–	15
Sesame oil, 1 tbsp		–	–	135	–	15
Soya oil, 1 tbsp		–	–	135	–	15
Stir-fry oil, 1 tbsp		–	–	135	–	15
Suet, shredded, 1 tbsp		–	–	124	–	13
Sunflower oil, 1 tbsp		–	–	124	–	13.8
Vegetable oil, 1 tbsp		–	–	135	–	15
Wheatgerm oil, 1 tbsp		–	–	135	–	15
For butter and margarine:						
see under Dairy						

TIP: Use chillies, garlic and herbs to flavour extra-virgin olive oil. Leave them to steep for a few days before use.

PASTA AND PIZZA

Although most pastas are low GI, they are high GL, meaning that an average portion will affect your blood sugar level, so you should combine them with low-GI sauces and opt for small-size portions. Wholewheat pasta is better for a GI regime as it contains more fibre. Egg pasta and filled pastas like ravioli have a higher fat content. Thin-crust pizzas with lots of vegetables on top are just about acceptable on a maintenance diet but not for weight loss. Study the nutrition label on ready-made pasta sauces as the sugar content may be high.

TIP: Choose vegetable-based sauces for pasta. Fresh tomatoes, spinach, broccoli, mushrooms or herbs are particularly good. Green or red pesto on penne with a green salad makes a simple low-GI meal.

Food type	GI	Carb (g)	Fibre (g)	Cal (kcal)	Pro (g)	Fat (g)
Pasta						
Dried lasagne sheets, cooked weight 100g:						
standard	●	18.1	–	89	3.1	0.4
verdi	●	18.3	–	93	3.2	0.4
Dried pasta shapes, cooked weight 100g:						
standard	●	18.1	–	89	3.1	0.4
verdi	●	18.3	–	93	3.2	0.4
Fresh egg pasta, 100g:						
conchiglie, penne, fusilli	●	31	1.4	170	7	2
lasagne sheets	●	29	4.6	150	6	1.1
spaghetti	●	23	1.6	135	6	2.1
tagliatelle	●	25	1.5	34	5	1.6
Macaroni, boiled, 100g	●	18.5	0.9	86	3	0.5
Spaghetti, cooked weight 100g:						
dried, egg	●	22.2	1.2	104	3.6	0.7
wholemeal	●	23.2	3.5	113	4.7	0.9
Stuffed fresh pasta, 100g:						
four cheese tortellini	●	20.1	0.9	133	5.6	3.3
spinach & ricotta tortellini verdi	●	21	2.4	149	6	4.5

TIP: Try different bases for 'pizzas': wholewheat pitta bread or a slice of sourdough or stoneground bread would work well. Top with plain tomato sauce and a few slices of mozzarella and olives.

Food type	GI	Carb (g)	Fibre (g)	Cal (kcal)	Pro (g)	Fat (g)
Stuffed fresh pasta, *contd:*						
ham & cheese tortellini	●	19.7	0.5	131	6.1	3.1
cheese & porcini ravioli	●	21.6	2.8	164	7.8	5.2
Pasta Sauces						
Amatriciana, fresh, low fat,						
100ml	●	6.3	1.2	50	2.3	1.9
Arrabbiata, fresh, low fat, 100ml	●	6.3	1.1	42	1.5	1.3
Bolognese, 100ml	●	2.5	0.6	161	11.8	11.6
Carbonara:						
fresh, 100ml	●	5.7	0.6	197	5.2	17.3
fresh, low fat, 100ml	●	5.5	0.6	97	4.8	6
Pesto:						
fresh, homemade, 100ml	●	6	1.4	45	2.2	1.3
green pesto, jar, 100ml	●	3.5	1.4	427	4.7	43.8
red pesto, jar, 100ml	●	3.1	0.4	358	4.1	36.6
Tomato & basil, fresh, 100ml	●	8.8	1.3	51	1.8	0.9
Canned Pasta						
Ravioli in tomato sauce,						
200g can	●	26	1.2	146	5.2	2.2
Spaghetti bolognese,						
200g can	●	25.6	1.4	172	6.8	4.6

TIP: Top a cooked pizza with fresh rocket for an authentic Italian finish.

Food type	GI	Carb (g)	Fibre (g)	Cal (kcal)	Pro (g)	Fat (g)
Spaghetti hoops, 200g	●	23.4	1.2	112	3.8	1.2
Spaghetti in tomato sauce, 200g can	●	26	1	122	3.4	0.4
diet, 200g	○	20.2	1.2	100	3.6	0.4
Spaghetti with sausages in tomato sauce, 200g	○	22	1	164	7.4	5.2
Spicy pepperoni pasta, 200g can	○	18.2	1	166	5.8	7.8
Spicy salsa twists, 200g	●	21.8	1.6	150	5.4	4.6
Pasta Ready Meals						
Bolognese shells Italiana, *diet*, per 100g	○	9.6	0.8	71	5.2	1.3
Canneloni bolognese, per 100g	○	11.8	n/a	149	6.1	8.3
Deep pasta bake, chicken & tomato, per 100g	○	13	1.3	95	4.5	3
Lasagne, each	●	46	n/a	440	24	18
vegetable, per 100g	○	12.6	0.9	110	5.3	4.7
Pasta bolognese, per 100g	●	54	n/a	375	18	9.6
Ravioli bianche, 100g	○	29.7	n/a	200	9.6	4.7

TIP: Cooked pasta shapes make a good basis for a summer raw vegetable salad. Make ribbons of courgette and carrot with a vegetable peeler and mix with a little vinaigrette dressing.

Food type	GI	Carb (g)	Fibre (g)	Cal (kcal)	Pro (g)	Fat (g)
Risotto, beef, per pack	●	57.8	5.6	346	15.3	5.9
Spaghetti bolognese, per pack	●	48	n/a	405	17	16
Pizza						
Cheese & onion deep filled pizza, 100g slice	●	30.3	1.3	223	8.4	8.2
Cheese & tomato pizza, 100g slice:	●	24.8	1.5	235	9	11.8
deep pan base	●	35.1	2.2	249	12.4	7.5
French bread base	●	31.4	–	230	10.6	7.8
thin base	○	33.9	1.9	277	14.4	10.3
French bread pizza, 100g slice	●	32.4	1.8	235	9.3	7.8
Ham & mushroom pizza, 100g slice	○	29.5	1.1	227	11.4	7.5
Pepperoni & sausage pizza, 100g slice	○	24.8	1.3	226	10.9	9.9
Pepperoni deep crust pizza, 100g slice	●	26.8	–	229	10.1	9
Pizza bases, 20cm diameter:						
deep pan	●	73	–	387	11	5.7
standard	●	72.8	–	387	11	5.7
stone baked	●	72.8	–	356	11	2.9

TIP: Don't overcook pasta. It should be *al dente* – with a bite to it – so that the digestive system has to work harder to break it down.

Food type	GI	Carb (g)	Fibre (g)	Cal (kcal)	Pro (g)	Fat (g)
Pizza topping, 100g:						
spicy tomato	●	9	1	66	1.6	2.6
tomato, cheese, onion & herbs	●	8.1	0.9	80	3	4
tomato, herbs & spices	●	9.4	0.8	67	1.5	2.6

For more pizzas: *see under*

Fast food

TIP: On a weight-loss diet, avoid canned pasta, gnocchi, pasta filled with cheese or meat, or sauces with added sugars such as sucrose. Opt for wholewheat pasta with light vegetable sauces and no added sugar.

PIES AND QUICHES

All the items in this section should be eaten only occasionally. Pastries of all types have high GI values, but you could lessen the blood sugar impact by choosing low-GI fillings and pies that just have pastry on top. Pork pies are made with a high-fat pastry, so are the least acceptable on a diet. Potato-topped pies like shepherd's and fish pies will have a slightly lower GI value than pastry-topped pies. If you are making your own, use sweet potato rather than ordinary potatoes.

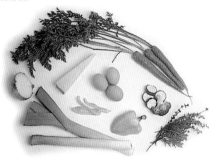

TIP: Pastry should only be eaten occasionally on a GI diet. Wholemeal is the slowest to convert to blood sugar and savoury fillings, especially vegetables, are the best options.

Food type	GI	Carb (g)	Fibre (g)	Cal (kcal)	Pro (g)	Fat (g)
Chicken & mushroom pie, individual	●	25.6	1.1	294	7.7	17.9
Cornish pasty, each	●	37.3	2.0	452	11.0	28.9
Game pie, 100g	●	34.7	1.3	381	12.2	22.5
Pastry, 100g cooked:						
flaky	●	45.9	1.4	560	5.6	40.6
shortcrust	●	54.2	2.2	521	6.6	32.3
wholemeal	●	44.6	6.3	499	8.9	32.9
Pork pie, individual	●	23.7	0.9	363	10.8	25.7
Quiche Lorraine, 100g:	●	19.6	0.7	358	13.7	25.5
cheese & egg, white pastry	●	17.3	0.6	314	12.5	22.2
cheese & egg, wholemeal pastry	●	14.5	1.9	308	13.2	22.4
Sausage rolls, each:						
flaky pastry	●	25.4	1	383	9.9	27.6
short pastry	●	19.4	0.8	289	11.1	19.3
Shepherd's pie, 100g	●	11	0.8	101	4.1	4.5
Steak & kidney pie, canned, 100g	●	13.3	–	154	8.7	8.1
Yorkshire pudding, each	●	5.5	0.2	47	1.5	1.8

TIP: For a quiche without a crust, cook your egg and cheese in a non-stick pan with some vegetables of choice to make a kind of frittata.

RICE AND NOODLES

Rice is either high or medium GI depending on the starches it contains and the way it has been processed. Easy-to-cook rices and the sticky, glutinous ones you are often served in Chinese, Thai and Japanese restaurants all have high GI values. Brown, basmati and long-grain rices are medium GI, as they contain a starch called amylose that it is harder for the digestive system to break down. Rice noodles are high GI and wheat noodles like soba and udon are medium GI. Cellophane noodles made from mung bean flour are the best choice on a GI diet.

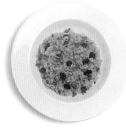

TIP: Basmati rice is the traditional curry rice. It has a unique nutty flavour and is one of the slowest rices to convert to blood sugar.

Food type	GI	Carb (g)	Fibre (g)	Cal (kcal)	Pro (g)	Fat (g)
Rice, cooked						
Arborio rice, 75g	●	23.3	0.3	105	2.2	0.3
Basmati rice, 75g	◐	22.7	–	103	2.7	0.2
Brown rice, 75g	◐	24	0.6	106	2	0.6
Egg fried rice, 75g	◐	19.2	0.3	156	2	8
Long grain rice, 75g	◐	22.6	–	103	2.1	0.3
Long grain & wild rice, 75g	◐	27.8	–	104	3.4	0.4
Pilau rice, 75g	◐	23	0.5	106	2.7	0.4
Pudding rice, 75g	●	24.2	0.2	107	1.9	0.3
Risotto rice, 75g	●	23.3	0.3	105	2.2	0.3
Short grain rice, 75g	●	26	0.7	108	2	0.3
White rice:						
plain, 75g	●	23.2	0.1	104	2	0.1
easy cook, 75g	●	23.2	0.1	104	2	0.1
Wholegrain rice, 75g	◐	21.2	0.6	102	2.7	0.7
Noodles, cooked						
Egg noodles, 75g	◐	9.8	0.5	47	2	0.4
Stir fry noodles, 75g	●	23.8	1.1	107	2.2	0.4
Thai rice noodles, 75g	●	26	0.7	108	2	0.3
Thread noodles, 75g	◐	7.4	–	51	1.8	1.5

TIP: Many noodles do not require cooking – just a short soak in boiling water. They can be combined with lots of stir-fried vegetables for a quick meal that is low-GI overall.

SNACKS, NIBBLES AND DIPS

Most GI diets recommend two or three snacks a day to prevent blood sugar dips between meals, but your choice of snack is all-important. Most crisps and nibbles are high in carbs, don't have any fibre and are coated with salt and artificial flavourings. They have a high GI content and should only be eaten rarely, in small quantities. Dried fruits vary in GI content. Dates are high, vine fruits and figs are medium and dried apricots are low. Ready-made dips can vary in GI count but hummus, guacamole and tzatziki are usually low.

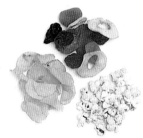

TIP: Seeds like sunflower and pumpkin are versatile as snacks and as salad ingredients. Roasted pumpkin seeds can also be sprinkled on top of soups instead of croutons.

Food type	GI	Carb (g)	Fibre (g)	Cal (kcal)	Pro (g)	Fat (g)
Crisps						
Cheese corn snacks,						
per pack (21g)	●	10.6	0.2	114	1.8	7.1
Hoop snacks, per pack (24g)	●	13.3	0.5	124	0.8	7.5
Potato crisps:						
cheese & onion,						
per pack (34.5g)	●	12.3	1.2	181	1.5	8.4
lightly salted, 25g	●	12.9	1.5	116.3	1.6	6.48
mature cheddar with chives, 25g	●	13.6	0.7	120	2	6.4
pickled onion, per pack (34.5g)	●	16.9	1.5	181	1.9	11.7
prawn cocktail,						
per pack (34.5g)	●	16.9	1.5	180	2	11.6
ready salted, per pack (34.5g)	●	17.2	1.6	186	1.9	12.2
roast chicken, (light),						
per pack (28g)	●	17.1	1.4	130	2.1	5.9
salsa with mesquite, 25g	●	13.5	1.4	115	1.5	1.5
salt & vinegar, per pack						
(34.5g)	●	16.7	1.5	180	1.9	11.7
salt & vinegar, (light),						
per pack (28g)	●	17.1	1.4	130	2.1	5.9

TIP: All the GI diets are full of ideas for healthy snacks, ranging from fresh fruit to high-fibre crispbreads, hazelnuts to low-fat yoghurts. You are advised to re-educate your palate away from the more salty and sugary snacks.

Food type	GI	Carb (g)	Fibre (g)	Cal (kcal)	Pro (g)	Fat (g)
Potato crisps, *contd:*						
sea salt with balsamic						
vinegar, 25g	●	15.2	1.1	117	1.5	6.1
smokey bacon, per pack (34.5g)	●	16.9	1.5	181	2	11.6
Quavers, per pack (20g)	●	12.1	0.2	103	0.6	5.8
Wheat crunchies:						
bacon flavour, per pack (35g)	●	17.3	0.8	152	3.4	7.7
salt & vinegar, per pack (35g)	●	19.1	0.9	170	3.7	8.7
spicy tomato, per pack (35g)	●	17.2	0.8	151	3.3	7.7
Worcester sauce, per pack (35g)	●	16.7	1.5	180	2	11.7
Nibbles						
Bombay mix, 50g	◐	19.2	3.1	262	8.2	17
Breadsticks, each	◐	3.6	0.2	21	0.6	0.4
Japanese rice crackers, 50g	●	39.9	0.2	199	4.5	2.3
Nachos, 100g	●	31	–	230	4	10
Olives, 15g black	◐	3.4	1.7	32	0.2	1.0
Peanuts & raisins, 50g	◐	18.8	2.2	218	7.7	13
yoghurt coated, 50g	●	24.9	0.9	245	4.9	13.8
Popcorn						
candied, 50g	●	38.8	–	240	1	10
plain, 50g	◐	24.3	–	296	3.1	21.4

TIP: Peanuts are low GI but choose the dry roast type rather than salted. See under Nuts and Seeds on page 163 for more information.

Food type	GI	Carb (g)	Fibre (g)	Cal (kcal)	Pro (g)	Fat (g)
Poppadums, each	○	11.2	2.6	70	5.3	0.4
fried in veg oil	○	9.8	–	92	4.3	4.2
spiced	○	11.4	2.6	70	5.1	0.5
Prawn crackers, 25g	●	15.5	0.3	132	0.1	7.7
Tortilla chips						
chilli flavour, 50g	●	32	–	248	3.5	13
cool original, per pack (40g)	●	25	1.4	204	3	10.5
jalapeño cheese flavour, 50g	●	30.5	–	260	3.5	13.5
pizza, per pack (40g)	●	23	1.4	202	3	11
salsa flavour, 50g	●	32.5	–	247	3.5	13
salted, 50g	●	30	2.5	230	3.8	11.3
tangy cheese, per pack (40g)	●	23	1.2	204	3.2	11
Trail mix, 50g	○	18.6	2.2	216	4.6	14.3
Twiglets, 50g	●	30	3.4	201	5.9	6.3
curry	●	28	3	225	4	10.7
tangy	●	28	2.8	227	4	2.8
Dried Fruit						
Apple rings, 25g	○	15	2.4	60	0.5	0.1
Apricots, 25g	○	15.5	2	60	1	0.1
Banana, 25g	○	13.4	2.5	55	0.8	0.2

TIP: Make your own dips using low-fat fromage frais, cream cheese or yoghurt as a base. Add spices, finely chopped vegetables or herbs to flavour.

Food type	GI	Carb (g)	Fibre (g)	Cal (kcal)	Pro (g)	Fat (g)
Banana chips, 25g	●	15	0.3	128	0.3	7.9
Currants, 25g	●	17	0.5	67	0.6	0.1
Dates, flesh & skin, 25g	●	17	1	68	0.8	0.1
Figs, 25g	●	13.2	1.9	57	0.9	0.4
Fruit salad, 25g	●	20.3	2	46	0.8	0.3
Mixed fruit, 25g	●	13.2	0.6	57	0.9	0.4
Pineapple, diced, 25g	●	17	2	69	0.6	0.3
Prunes, 25g	●	8.4	3.4	34	0.5	–
Raisins, seedless, 25g	●	17.3	0.5	68	0.5	0.1
Sultanas, 25g	●	17.3	0.5	69	0.7	0.1
Nuts and Seeds						
Almonds:						
weighed with shells, 50g	●	1.3	1.4	115	5.2	5.2
flaked/ground, 25g	●	1.7	1.8	153	5.3	14
Brazils:						
weighed with shells, 50g	●	0.7	1.9	157	3.3	15.7
kernel only, 25g	●	0.8	2	171	3.5	17
Cashews:						
kernel only, 25g	●	4.7	0.8	152	5.1	12.7
pieces, 25g	●	4.3	0.8	156	6	12.7

TIP: Snacks made from maize, like tortilla chips, have a lower GI than potato crisps but they're still in the 'red' category. Dip them in low-GI guacamole to lower the overall GI value of the snack.

Food type	GI	Carb (g)	Fibre (g)	Cal (kcal)	Pro (g)	Fat (g)
Chestnuts, kernel only, 25g	●	9.2	1	43	0.5	0.7
Coconut: *see under* Fruit						
Hazelnuts:						
weighed with shell, 50g	●	1.2	1.3	124	1.4	6
kernel only, 25g	●	1.5	1.6	163	3.5	15.9
Hickory nuts: *see* Pecans						
Macadamia nuts, salted, 50g	●	2.4	2.7	374	4	2.7
Mixed nuts, 25g	●	2	1.5	152	5.7	13.5
Monkey nuts: *see* Peanuts						
Peanuts:						
plain, weighed with shells, 50g	●	4.3	2	195	8.9	15.9
plain, kernel only, 25g	●	6.3	3.1	141	6.4	11.5
dry roasted, 50g	●	5.2	3.2	295	12.8	2
roasted & salted, 50g	●	3.6	3	301	12.3	26.5
Pecans, kernel only, 25g	●	1.5	1.2	172	2.3	17.5
Pine nuts, kernel only, 25g	●	1	0.5	172	3.5	17.2
Pistachios, weighed with shells, 50g	●	2.3	1.7	83	2.5	7.7
Poppy seeds, 10g	●	1.9	–	56	2	4.4
Pumpkin seeds, 25g	●	11.8	1.1	143	7.3	12
Sesame seeds, 10g	●	0.6	0.7	64	2.3	5.8
Sunflower seeds, 25g	●	4.7	3	149	5.9	11.9

TIP: Drain and rinse a small can of kidney beans and mash together with tomato juice and grated onion for a Mexican-style dip.

Food type	GI	Carb (g)	Fibre (g)	Cal (kcal)	Pro (g)	Fat (g)
Walnuts:						
weighed with shell, 50g	●	0.7	0.8	148	3.2	14.7
halves , 25g	●	0.8	0.9	172	3.7	17.1
Dips						
Curry & mango dip, 100g	●	6.1	–	334	4.5	32.4
Mexican dips, 100g:						
guacamole	●	0.6	0.1	159	1.2	16
Mexican bean	●	12.1	2.4	89	2.7	3.3
spicy	●	4.8	–	324	4.7	31.7
Hummus, 100g	●	11.6	2.4	187	7.6	12.6
Onion & chive dip, 100g	●	2.1	–	341	4.6	34.9
Salsa, 100g						
cheese	●	9.3	–	143	2.5	10.7
cool, organic	●	6.3	1.2	141	1.2	0.4

TIP: There are several tricks that will help you keep to your GI diet at a party. First of all, eat a good, steady-fuel-providing meal before you leave; this will help to stop cravings and stop you absorbing alcohol so quickly. Instead of dipping bread and crackers into dips, choose vegetable crudités; instead of sausage rolls, choose cocktail sausages on their own, or chicken drumsticks if available; drink white wine spritzers instead of gin and tonic or sparkling wine. And remember that salsa and tzatziki are much lower in calories than creamy dips like taramasalata, even if they are all in the low-GI category.

Food type	GI	Carb (g)	Fibre (g)	Cal (kcal)	Pro (g)	Fat (g)
Salsa, *contd:*						
hot, organic	●	6.2	1.1	141	1.1	0.4
picante	●	4.6	–	28	1.4	0.5
Sour-cream based dips, 100g	●	4	–	360	2.9	37
Taramasalata, 100g	●	7.4	1.8	523	2.7	53.6
Tzatziki, 100g	●	1.9	0.3	66	3.8	4.9

TIP: Reading the labels is all-important when it comes to snacks, as the salt and fat content can be very high. If there is more than 0.25g of salt (or 0.2g of sodium) per 100g of snack, then it is particularly salty. If there is more than 5g of fat (or more than 2g of saturated fat) per 100g, choose something else instead.

SOUP

Soups can make an ideal lunch on a GI diet but beware of cream-based ones or those labelled 'cream of...'. If you are buying a can or carton, read the ingredients list to see how high the soup is in sugars, gums and flour or cornflour thickeners. Clear consommés and thick vegetable and bean soups are both low GI. Ingredients to avoid are root vegetables like parsnip and carrot, rice, pasta and cream. Try to eat soup without bread on the side or croutons sprinkled on top.

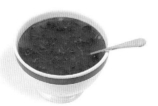

TIP: A can of consommé makes a low-GI base for soup. Add a spoonful or so of grated or thinly sliced raw vegetables like carrot or celery or even grated orange zest just before serving.

Food type	GI	Carb (g)	Fibre (g)	Cal (kcal)	Pro (g)	Fat (g)
Canned Soups						
Beef broth, 200ml	●	13.6	1.4	82	4	1.2
Beef consommé, 200ml	●	1.4	–	26	4.8	–
Beef & vegetable soup, 200ml	●	14.6	1.8	90	4.8	1.4
Broccoli soup, 200ml	●	11.8	0.8	90	2.6	3.6
Broccoli & potato soup, 200ml	●	11.6	1.4	62	2.6	0.6
Carrot & butter bean soup, 200ml	●	15.8	3.8	110	3.2	3.8
Carrot & coriander soup, 200ml	●	12.4	1.2	104	1.4	5.4
Carrot & lentil soup, low calorie, 200ml	●	12	1.6	62	2.8	0.2
Carrot, parsnip & nutmeg organic, 200ml	●	11.4	2	54	1.4	0.4
Chicken broth, 200ml	●	10.6	1.2	68	2.4	1.8
Chicken soup, low calorie, 200ml	●	8.2	–	60	2.4	2
Chicken & ham, 200ml	●	13.8	1.4	92	4.3	2
low calorie	●	8.8	0.9	59	1.1	2.2
Chicken & sweetcorn soup, 200ml	●	12.4	1.2	78	3.2	1.8
Chicken & vegetable soup, 200ml	●	11.2	3.2	62	2.6	1

TIP: 200ml of soup will fill the average soup bowl three-quarters full. Sachets of soup mixed with boiling water fill a mug of around 250ml.

Food type	GI	Carb (g)	Fibre (g)	Cal (kcal)	Pro (g)	Fat (g)
Chicken & white wine soup, 200ml	●	8	–	98	2	6.6
Chicken noodle soup, low calorie, 200ml	○	6.2	0.4	32	1.4	0.2
Cock-a-leekie soup, 200ml	○	8	0.6	58	1.8	2
Consommé, 200ml	○	1	–	14	2.6	–
Cream of asparagus, 200ml	●	11.6	0.4	132	2.2	8.6
Cream of celery soup, 200ml	●	6.4	–	94	1.2	6.8
Cream of chicken soup, 200ml	●	7	–	96	2.2	7.2
Cream of chicken & mushroom, 200ml	●	7	–	112	1.8	8.8
Cream of mushroom, 200ml	●	10.6	–	138	3.4	9
Cream of tomato, 200ml	●	21.2	1.4	142	3	5
Creamy chicken with vegetables, fresh soup, 200ml	●	11	0.8	194	3.8	15
Cullen skink, 200ml	●	15.4	0.6	178	12.2	7.4
French onion soup, 200ml	○	8.4	0.8	44	1.4	0.4
Garden pea & mint fresh soup, 200ml	●	12.2	3	124	4.6	6.4
Italian bean & pasta soup, 200ml	○	14	2.6	76	3.8	0.4
Lentil soup, 200ml	○	8.6	–	54	2.6	1.2

TIP: Add beans, lentils or pearl barley to your homemade soups to lower their GI value.

Food type	GI	Carb (g)	Fibre (g)	Cal (kcal)	Pro (g)	Fat (g)
Lobster bisque, 200ml	●	9.4	0.4	102	6.8	4.2
Mediterranean tomato, 200ml	◐	13.8	1.4	66	2	0.4
Minestrone soup:						
chunky fresh, 200ml	◐	14	2.4	84	3.4	1.6
Miso, 200ml	●	47	–	406	26.6	12.4
Mulligatawny beef curry soup						
200ml	◐	14.4	1	120	3.6	5.4
Mushroom soup:						
low calorie, 200ml	◐	10	0.2	64	2.6	1.4
Oxtail soup, 200ml	●	10.6	–	80	2.8	3
Parsnip & carrot:						
low calorie, 200ml	◐	10.6	1.8	50	1	0.4
Pea & ham, 200ml	●	16.2	2.4	116	5.8	3.2
Potato & leek, 200ml	◐	12.6	1	80	2	2.4
Royal game, 200ml	◐	11	0.8	72	4.8	1
Scotch broth, 200ml	●	14.2	1.8	94	3.8	2.4
Spicy parsnip, 200ml	●	12.2	3	102	2.2	5
Spicy tomato & rice with						
sweetcorn, 200ml	●	18.4	1.2	90	2.6	0.6
Spring vegetable soup, 200ml	◐	9	–	42	1	0.2

TIP: Lift a basic soup to haute cuisine with a special garnish – a swirl of oil-thinned pesto on a tomato soup; chopped herbs on a mushroom soup; or a chilli-flavoured sherry in any soup (steep a dried chilli in a little dry sherry for at least a week).

Food type	GI	Carb (g)	Fibre (g)	Cal (kcal)	Pro (g)	Fat (g)
Thai chicken with noodles, 200ml	●	13.6	0.6	94	3.4	0.8
Tomato soup:						
low calorie, 200ml	●	9.4	0.6	52	1.4	1.0
Vegetable soup, 200ml	●	12.4	–	70	1.6	1.6
chunky fresh, 200ml	●	15.6	2.2	78	3.2	0.4
low calorie, 200ml	●	11.8	1.8	62	2	0.6
Winter vegetable soup, 200ml	●	16.4	2.2	92	5.6	0.4
low calorie, 200ml	●	12.0	1.6	62	3.2	0.2
Sachet/Cup Soups						
Beef & tomato cup soup, per sachet	●	15.5	1	71	1.3	0.4
Broccoli & cauliflower:						
thick & creamy, per sachet	●	17.2	0.6	120	1.9	4.8
low calorie, per sachet	●	10.3	0.4	59	1.1	1.5
Cajun spicy vegetable low calorie soup, per sachet	●	10.3	1.1	58	1.6	1.3
Cheese & broccoli cup soup, per sachet	●	23.5	1.9	160	5.2	5

TIP: For a refreshing chilled summer soup, whizz together two peeled and deseeded cucumbers, a few mint leaves and 200ml vegetable stock with 100g no-fat plain yoghurt. Refrigerate and season with salt to taste. Serve garnished with a whole mint leaf.

Food type	GI	Carb (g)	Fibre (g)	Cal (kcal)	Pro (g)	Fat (g)
Chicken soup, cup soup						
per sachet	●	12.4	0.6	98	1.5	4.7
Chicken & leek cup soup,						
per sachet	●	14.1	0.7	154	2.4	3.6
Chicken & mushroom						
per sachet:	●	20.2	1.3	132	3.7	4
low calorie	●	8.8	0.9	59	1.1	2.2
Chicken & sweetcorn soup:						
low calorie, per sachet	●	9.2	0.3	59	1.2	1.9
Chicken noodle soup:						
Batchelors cup soup, sachet	●	15.1	0.8	182	7.2	3.8
Chicken, noodle & vegetable:						
low calorie, per sachet	●	10.2	0.7	59	1.6	1.4
Chinese chicken cup soup						
per sachet	●	19.1	2	101	3.5	1.2
Cream of asparagus cup soup,						
per sachet	●	19.9	1.1	133	2.1	5
Cream of chicken & vegetable,						
cup soup, per sachet	●	18	0.6	113	2.1	5.9
Cream of mushroom, cup soup						
per sachet	●	15.4	0.7	129	1.2	6.6

TIP: For a 'cream soup' effect without the cream, purée cooked cannellini beans or chickpeas and add them to your stock and vegetables. Use red beans, such as kidney beans, in a tomato-based soup.

Food type	GI	Carb (g)	Fibre (g)	Cal (kcal)	Pro (g)	Fat (g)
Cream of vegetable cup soup, per sachet	●	19.8	1.2	144	1.9	6.3
Creamy potato & leek cup soup, per sachet	●	20.9	3.2	133	2.3	4.4
Golden vegetable:						
cup soup, per sachet	●	15.3	0.9	70	1	0.5
low calorie, per sachet	●	9.7	1.5	58	1.1	1.7
Hot & sour cup soup, sachet	●	18.7	1.2	91	2.5	0.7
Leek & potato low calorie, per sachet	●	10.2	0.5	57	0.9	1.4
Mediterranean tomato:						
low calorie per sachet	●	9.6	0.7	58	1.1	1.7
Minestrone soup:						
cup soup, per sachet	●	17.9	1.1	100	1.9	2.3
low calorie, per sachet	●	9.3	0.7	54	1.3	1.3
Oxtail soup, per sachet	●	13.7	1	76	1.5	1.7

TIP: Tuscan bean soup is a classic low-GI dish. For a quick and easy version, sauté 2 onions, 2 celery stalks, 1 leek, 6 cloves of garlic and a teaspoon of oregano and basil in a little olive oil. When they are soft and the onion is translucent (about 10 minutes), add a 400g can of tomatoes, 250ml of boiling water or vegetable stock and some chopped fresh parsley. Simmer for 5 minutes then add a can of mixed beans and leave them to heat through. Season to taste and serve with finely chopped peppers and onion sprinkled on top.

Food type	GI	Carb (g)	Fibre (g)	Cal (kcal)	Pro (g)	Fat (g)
Spicy vegetable cup soup, per sachet	●	22.3	1.2	109	2.9	1
Tomato cup soup, per sachet	●	17.3	1.2	85	0.8	1.4
Tomato & vegetable cup soup, per sachet	●	18.6	1	109	2.6	2.7

TIP: Add nuts and seeds to your soups to give them better texture and to provide some extra vitamins and minerals. Sprinkle pumpkin, sunflower, flax, poppy or hemp seeds on top, or use ground almonds stirred through to thicken your soup.

SUGAR AND SWEETENERS

Sugars are a flashing red light area. They should be avoided as much as possible on any kind of weight-loss diet. Gradually reduce the sugar used in tea or coffee, forego puddings, biscuits and confectionery and you should start losing weight. Two types of sugar in particular – glucose and maltose – are high GI and you should check for them on ingredients lists. Artificial sweeteners still carry a health stigma although some nutritionists think that the sugar-based Splenda is the best alternative so far.

TIP: If you don't want to use artificial sweeteners, try fructose, a fruit sugar that is sold as granules. It has a GI rating of 23 (low), while white sugar is 65 (medium). You use fructose just as you would sugar, except that it is about a third sweeter, so you don't need as much.

Food type	GI	Carb (g)	Fibre (g)	Cal (kcal)	Pro (g)	Fat (g)
Amber sugar crystals, 1 tsp	●	4.9	–	20	–	–
Date syrup, 1 tsp	●	3.6	–	15	–	–
Golden syrup, 1 tsp	●	4	–	15	–	–
Honey, 1 tsp	●	5.8	–	21	–	–
Icing sugar, 1 tsp	●	5	–	20	–	–
Jaggery	●	4.9	–	18	–	–
Maple syrup, 1 tsp	●	3.4	–	13	–	–
Molasses, 1 tsp	●	4	–	16	–	–
Sugar:						
caster, 1 tsp	●	4.9	–	20	–	–
dark brown, soft, 1 tsp	●	4.7	–	19	–	–
demerara, cane, 1 tsp	●	5	–	20	–	–
granulated, 1 tsp	●	5	–	20	–	–
light brown, soft, 1 tsp	●	4.8	–	19	–	–
preserving, 1 tsp	●	4.9	–	20	–	–
cube, white, each	●	4.9	–	20	–	–
Treacle, black, 1 tsp	●	3.4	–	12.9	–	–
Sweeteners						
Canderel, 1 tsp	●	0.47	–	1.9	0.01	–
Hermesetas, 1 tsp	●	0.28	0.21	1.4	0.01	–
Splenda, 1 tsp	●	0.5	–	2	–	–

TIP: Always check ingredients labels to search out the hidden sugars in foods (see 'Reading Labels', page 30).

SWEETS AND CHOCOLATES

You won't find any green lights in this section. Sugar levels vary in different types of sweets but when you read the ingredients label sugar will invariably be at the top of the list, meaning it is the main one. Chocolate with a high cocoa content (at least 60%) has less sugar and saturated fat than other forms of sweets, so you could allow yourself a couple of squares for a treat from time to time. Nuts will help to slow the absorption of sugars, and chocolate Brazil nuts are a good source of the mineral selenium.

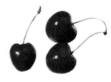

TIP: Chewing gums don't have a GI value, but they do use artificial sweeteners and some contain phenylalanine, excessive consumption of which can have a laxative effect.

Food type	GI	Carb (g)	Fibre (g)	Cal (kcal)	Pro (g)	Fat (g)
After Dinner Mints:						
dark chocolate, 25g	●	18.2	0.3	104	0.6	3.2
white chocolate, 25g	●	19.2	–	106	0.7	2.9
American Hard Gums, 25g	●	21.4	–	86.3	–	–
Barley Sugar, 25g	●	24.3	–	97.3	–	–
Black Jack chews, 25g	●	28.3	–	99.8	0.2	1.5
Blue Riband, 25g	●	16	0.3	129	1.3	6.7
Bonbons, 25g:						
buttermints	●	21.5	–	106	0.2	2.2
lemon	●	21.4	–	104.3	0.3	1.9
strawberry	●	103.8	0.2	104	0.3	1.9
toffee	●	20.4	–	108	0.4	2.7
Bounty, 25g:						
dark chocolate	●	14.4	–	120	0.8	0.6
milk chocolate	●	14.1	–	121	1.2	6.7
Breakaway, 25g	●	14.9	1.2	124	1.7	6.4
Buttermints, 25g	●	22.2	–	101	–	0.9
Butterscotch, 25g	●	22.5	–	103	–	1.4
Chocolate buttons, 25g	●	14.2	–	131	2	7.4
Caramel chocolate bar, 25g	●	13.6	–	141	1.5	9
Caramels, milk & plain chocolate, 25g	●	24.1	–	123	–	–

TIP: If you get a sweet craving, nibble some seedless grapes, dried apricots or cherries. Cherries have the lowest GI rating of any fruits.

Food type	GI	Carb (g)	Fibre (g)	Cal (kcal)	Pro (g)	Fat (g)
Chewing gum:						
Airwaves, sugarfree , 5g		–	–	7.6	–	–
Doublemint, 5g		–	–	15.4	–	–
Extra peppermint, 5g		–	–	8.2	–	–
Ice White, sugarfree, 5g		–	–	9.8	–	–
Juicy Fruit, 5g		–	–	14.8	–	–
Peppermint, sugarfree, 5g		–	–	9.8	–	–
Spearmint, sugarfree, 5g		–	–	9.6	–	–
Chocolate cream, 25g	●	17.2	–	106	0.7	3.9
Chocolate éclairs, 25g	●	18	0.1	120	0.7	5
Chocolate limes, 25g	●	22.7	0.1	102	0.2	4.7
Chocolate Orange, 25g:						
dark chocolate	●	14.2	1.6	128	1	7.3
milk chocolate	●	14.5	0.5	132	2	7.4
Chocolate Truffles, 25g:						
with coffee liqueur	●	15.9	0.1	119	1	5.6
with orange liqueur	●	15.8	0.1	119	1	5.6
with whiskey cream	●	15.9	0.1	119	1	5.6
Chocolate, 25g:						
milk	●	14.9	–	132	2.1	7.6
plain	●	16.2	–	131	1.2	7.3

TIP: Plain dark chocolate (60% cocoa solids or more) contains far less sugar than milk or white chocolate. Added nuts or dried fruit lower the GI even more.

Food type	GI	Carb (g)	Fibre (g)	Cal (kcal)	Pro (g)	Fat (g)
Chocolate, contd:						
white	●	14.6	–	132	2	7.7
raisin & biscuit	●	15.1	–	122	1.5	6
fruit & nut	●	13.9	–	122	2	6.6
wholenut	●	12.2	–	138	2.3	8.8
Coolmints, 25g	●	24.7	–	59	–	–
Cough candy, 25g	●	23.8	–	95.8	–	–
Cream toffees, assorted, 25g	●	18.3	–	108	0.9	3.5
Cream eggs, 25g	●	17.9	–	111	0.8	4
Crunchie, 25g	●	18	–	116	1	4.5
Dairy toffee, 25g	●	18.8	–	118	0.5	4.6
Double Decker, 25g	●	16.2	–	116	1.3	5.2
Energy Tablets, 25g						
glucose	●	22.3	–	90	–	–
orange	●	22.2	–	90	–	–
lemon	●	22.2	–	90	–	–
Everton mints, 25g	●	22.5	–	103	0.2	1.4
Flake bar, 25g	●	13.9	–	133	2	7.7
Fruit gums, 25g	●	20.2	–	86	1.2	–
Fruit pastilles, 25g	●	20.9	–	88	1.1	–
Fudge, 25g	●	18	–	111	0.7	4.1

TIP: Dip strawberries into a bowl of melted high-cocoa chocolate for an occasional after-dinner treat. Experiment with other low-GI fruits as well – pears or apples work well.

Food type	GI	Carb (g)	Fibre (g)	Cal (kcal)	Pro (g)	Fat (g)
Galaxy (Mars), 25g:						
chocolate	◐	14.2	–	133	2.3	7.5
caramel	●	15	–	122	1.3	6.3
double nut & raisin	◐	13.9	–	134	13.9	7.7
hazelnut	◐	12.1	–	143	1.9	9.7
praline	◐	13	–	145	1.3	9.9
Jellies, assorted, 25g	●	20.4	–	77	–	–
Kit Kat, 25g:						
4-finger	●	15.4	0.3	127	1.5	6.6
Chunky	●	15.3	0.2	129	1.4	6.9
Lion Bar, 25g	●	16.9	–	122	1.2	5.6
Liquorice Allsorts, 25g	●	13.8	0.4	88	0.6	1.1
Lockets, 25g	●	24	0.3	96	–	–
M & Ms, 25g:						
chocolate	◐	17.4	–	122	1.2	5.3
peanut	◐	14.3	–	128	2.6	6.8
Maltesers, 25g	●	15.4	–	124	2.5	5.8
Mars Bar, 25g	●	17.3	–	112	1	4.4
Minstrels, 25g	●	17.4	–	123	1.5	5.3
Milky Way, 25g	●	17.9	–	113	1.1	4.2
Mint Crisp, 25g	●	17.6	–	126	1.6	5.6
Mint humbugs, 25g	●	22.4	–	103	0.2	1.5

TIP: Rick Gallop's Chocolate Drop Cookies use a purée of white kidney beans to provide fibre, making a green-light, low-GI chocolate treat.

Food type	GI	Carb (g)	Fibre (g)	Cal (kcal)	Pro (g)	Fat (g)
Mint imperials, 25g	●	24.5	–	99	0.1	–
Munchies, 25g:						
original	●	15.9	0.1	123	1.2	6
mint	●	16.9	0.4	108	1	4.1
Murray Mints, 25g	●	22.6	–	102	–	1.3
Orange Cream, 25g	●	17.2	–	106	0.7	3.9
Peanut Lion Bar, 25g	●	14.2	–	131	1.8	7.4
Pear Drops, 25g	●	23.9	–	96	–	–
Peppermints, 25g	●	25.6	–	98	0.1	0.2
Peppermint Cream, 25g	●	17.2	–	106	0.7	3.9
Picnic, 25g	●	14.9	–	119	1.9	5.7
Pineapple chunks, 25g	●	23.8	–	96	–	–
Polos:						
mints, 25g	●	24.6	–	101	–	2.5
sugar-free, 25g	●	24.8	–	60	–	–
smoothies, 25g	●	22.1	–	103	–	1.7
Pontefract cakes, 25g	●	16.7	0.6	70	0.6	0.1
Poppets, 25g:						
peanut	●	9.3	–	136	–	9.3
raisins	●	16.5	–	102	–	3.5
Refreshers, 25g	●	22.6	–	94	–	0.1
Revels, 25g	●	16.4	–	124	1.6	5.8

TIP: Note that the 25g serving size given for sweets and chocolate in this section is the size of the very smallest bars, not the family-size ones.

Food type	GI	Carb (g)	Fibre (g)	Cal (kcal)	Pro (g)	Fat (g)
Ripple, 25g	●	14.2	–	133	2.3	7.5
Rolo, 25g	●	17.1	0.1	118	0.8	5.1
Sherbet Lemons, 25g	●	23.5	–	96	–	–
Snickers, 25g	●	13.8	–	128	2.6	6.9
Softfruits, 25g	●	22	–	92	–	0.3
Softmints, 25g	●	22	–	94	–	0.6
Spearmints, Extra Strong, 25g	●	24.7	–	99	0.1	–
Sugared almonds, 25g	●	19.5	0.6			
Sweet peanuts, 25g	●	20	0.4	107	0.8	0.4
Sweets, boiled, 25g	●	21.8	–	82	–	–
Toblerone, 25g	●	14.8	0.6	131	1.4	7.4
Toffees, mixed, 25g	●	17.8	–	108	0.5	4.3
Toffee Crisp, 25g	●	15.1	0.2	128	1.1	7
Toffo, 25g	●	17.5	–	113	0.6	4.6
Topic, 25g	●	14.2	–	123	1.2	6.7
Tunes, 25g	●	24.5	–	98	–	–
Turkish Delight, 25g	●	18.3	–	91	0.5	1.8
Twix, 25g	●	15.9	–	124	1.5	6

TIP: Make your own chocolate pistachio nuts. Microwave 12 squares of dark chocolate for 2 minutes on high and stir until completely melted. Shell and toast 150g of pistachio nuts. Stir the nuts into the chocolate, spoon the mixture onto a greaseproof paper-lined baking tin then place in the fridge for an hour. Each 25g serving will have 150 calories and 10g fat, but it's just medium on the GI scale.

Food type	GI	Carb (g)	Fibre (g)	Cal (kcal)	Pro (g)	Fat (g)
Walnut whip, vanilla, 25g	●	15.2	–	124	1.5	6.4
Wine gums 25g	●	19	–	84	1.5	–

TIP: Don't beat yourself up if you slip up from time to time. Many diet experts advise that you follow the 80:20 rule – keep to the diet 80% of the time and indulge yourself not more than 20% of the time.

VEGETABLES

No fresh vegetable should be ignored on the GI diet but some are better than others. The watery ones – salad leaves, cabbage, spinach, courgettes, onions and garlic – have the lowest GI value. Mushrooms and aubergines are also low GI. Carrots, tomatoes and peas are slightly higher but contain valuable nutrients so shouldn't be avoided. The starchiest root vegetables like parsnips, beetroot, potatoes and the winter squashes should be eaten in moderation.

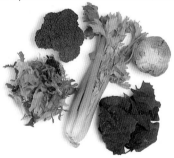

TIP: Sweet potatoes have a lower GI than ordinary potatoes and can be cooked in the same way. Try making Shepherds' Pie with a mashed sweet potato topping or serving baked sweet potatoes with a chilli bean topping.

Food type	GI	Carb (g)	Fibre (g)	Cal (kcal)	Pro (g)	Fat (g)
Artichokes, 1 globe	●	2.7	–	18	2.8	0.2
Artichoke, Jerusalem, boiled, 90g	●	9.5	–	37	1.4	0.1
Asparagus, 6 spears, boiled	●	3.8	1.5	21	2.4	0.3
Aubergine, half medium, fried	●	1.4	0.5	151	0.6	16
Avocado, half	●	8	3.4	160	1.9	14
Bamboo shoots, raw, 75g	●	0.5	1.3	8.2	1.1	0.5
Beans, broad, boiled, 75g	●	4.2	4.0	36	3.8	0.6
Beans, French, 100g boiled	●	2.9	2.4	22	1.8	0.5
Beans, runner, 50g, trimmed, boiled	●	1.1	1.5	9	0.6	0.2
Beansprouts, mung, 25g:						
raw	●	2	0.75	7.8	0.7	0.1
stirfried in blended oil	●	0.6	0.2	18	0.5	1.5
Beetroot, 90g:						
pickled	●	5.0	1.5	25	1.1	0.2
boiled	●	8.6	1.7	41	2.0	0.1
Broccoli, florets, boiled, 60g	●	0.6	1.4	14	1.9	0.5
Brussels sprouts, 6 trimmed, boiled	●	10.9	3.3	49	3.3	0.6

TIP: Canned vegetables lose their vitamin C content during processing but frozen vegetables, which are generally processed soon after picking, have a similar nutrition profile to fresh.

Food type	GI	Carb (g)	Fibre (g)	Cal (kcal)	Pro (g)	Fat (g)
Cabbage (Savoy, Summer), 75g:						
trimmed	●	3.1	1.8	20	1.3	0.3
shredded & boiled	●	1.9	1.6	14	0.6	0.4
Spring greens, raw	●	2.3	2.5	25	2.3	0.7
Spring greens, boiled	●	1.2	1.9	15	1.4	0.5
white	●	3.7	1.6	20	1.0	0.2
Carrot:						
1 medium, raw	●	7.9	2.4	35	0.6	0.3
1 medium, raw (young)	●	6.9	2.7	34	0.8	2.7
grated, 40g	●	3.2	0.9	15	0.2	0.1
boiled (frozen), 80g	●	3.8	1.8	18	0.3	0.2
boiled (young), 80g	●	3.5	1.8	18	0.5	0.3
Cassava, 100g:						
baked	●	40.1	1.7	155	0.7	0.2
boiled	●	33.5	1.4	130	0.5	0.2
Cauliflower, 100g:						
raw	●	3.0	1.8	34	3.6	0.9
boiled	●	2.1	1.6	28	2.9	0.9
Celeriac, 100g:						
flesh only, raw	●	2.3	3.7	18	1.2	0.4
flesh only, boiled	●	1.9	3.2	15	0.9	0.5

TIP: You can grow your own salad ingredients in a garden or window-box. Lettuce, tomatoes, cucumber, radishes and cress are all easy to grow from seed.

Food type	GI	Carb (g)	Fibre (g)	Cal (kcal)	Pro (g)	Fat (g)
Celery, 100g:						
stem only, raw	●	0.9	1.1	7	0.5	0.2
stem only, boiled	●	0.8	1.2	8	0.5	0.3
Chicory, 100g	●	2.8	0.9	11	0.5	0.6
Corn-on-the-cob						
boiled, 1 medium cob	●	22.4	2.5	127	4.8	2.6
mini corncobs, boiled, 100g	●	2.7	2.0	24	2.5	0.4
See also: Sweetcorn						
Courgettes (zucchini):						
trimmed, 50g	●	0.9	0.4	9	0.9	0.2
trimmed, boiled, 75g	●	1.5	0.9	14	1.5	0.3
trimmed, sliced, 75g	●					
fried in corn oil, 75g	●	1.9	0.9	47	1.9	3.6
Cucumber, trimmed, 75g	●	1.1	0.4	7.5	0.5	0.1
Eggplant: *see* Aubergine						
Fennel, Florence						
boiled, 75g	●	1.1	1.7	8	0.7	0.1
Garlic, half tsp purée or						
1 clove, crushed	●	1.9	0.9	60	0.1	5.7
Gherkins,						
pickled, 75g	●	1.9	0.9	10	0.7	0.08
Ginger root, half tsp, grated	●	–	5	0.2	–	

TIP: Eat vegetables raw, so that nutrients aren't lost in cooking. Try mixing grated carrot and thinly sliced courgette with some raisins.

Food type	GI	Carb (g)	Fibre (g)	Cal (kcal)	Pro (g)	Fat (g)
Greens, spring: *see* Cabbage						
Gumbo: *see* Okra						
Kale, curly, 40g:						
raw	●	0.6	1.2	13	1.4	0.6
shredded, boiled	●	0.4	1.1	10	0.9	0.4
Kohlrabi, 85g:						
raw	●	3.1	1.9	20	1.4	0.2
boiled	●	2.6	1.6	15	1.0	0.2
Ladies' Fingers: *see* Okra						
Leeks:						
trimmed, 60g	●	1.7	1.3	13	1.0	0.3
chopped, boiled, 100g	●	2.6	1.7	21	1.2	0.7
Lettuce, 1 cup (30g):						
green	●	0.5	0.3	4	0.2	0.1
iceberg	●	0.6	0.2	4	0.2	0.1
mixed leaf	●	0.8	0.8	5	0.4	0.03
Mediterranean salad leaves	●	0.8	0.3	4.5	0.3	0.1
spinach, rocket & watercress	●	0.4	0.4	7.5	0.9	0.3
Mange-tout, 50g:						
raw	●	2.1	1.6	16	1.8	0.1
boiled	●	1.6	1.1	13	1.6	0.05
stir-fried	●	1.8	1.2	36	1.9	2.4

TIP: Choose a rainbow mix of vegetables and stir fry, flavoured with garlic, ginger and soy sauce, for a colourful and nutritious dish.

Food type	GI	Carb (g)	Fibre (g)	Cal (kcal)	Pro (g)	Fat (g)
Marrow:						
flesh only, 50g	●	1.1	0.2	6	0.2	0.1
flesh only, boiled, 75g	●	1.2	0.5	7	0.3	0.1
Mooli: see Radish, white						
Mushrooms, common, 40g:						
raw	●	0.2	0.4	5	0.7	0.2
boiled	●	0.2	0.4	4	0.7	0.1
fried in oil	●	0.1	0.6	63	1	6.5
canned	●	–	0.2	4	0.8	0.2
Mushrooms, oyster, 30g	●	–	–	2	0.5	0.06
Mushrooms, shiitake:						
boiled, 40g	●	4.9	n/a	22	0.6	0.1
dried, 20g	●	12.8	n/a	59	1.9	0.2
Neeps (Scotland): see Swede						
Okra (gumbo, ladies' fingers):						
raw, 25g	●	0.8	1.0	8	0.7	0.2
boiled, 30g	●	0.8	1.0	8	0.7	0.2
stir-fried, 30g	●	1.3	1.9	81	1.3	7.8
Onions:						
raw, flesh only, 30g	●	2.4	0.4	11	0.4	0.1
boiled, 40g	●	1.5	0.3	7	0.2	–
cocktail, drained, 40g	●	1.2	n/a	6	0.2	–

TIP: Portion sizes are roughly half a cup, unless otherwise stated. Gram weights are also given, since some would be tricky to fit in a cup.

Food type	GI	Carb (g)	Fibre (g)	Cal (kcal)	Pro (g)	Fat (g)
Onions, *contd:*						
fried in vegetable oil, 40g	●	5.6	1.2	66	0.9	4.5
pickled, drained, 40g	●	2.0	0.5	10	0.4	0.1
Parsnips, trimmed, peeled,						
boiled, 80g	●	10.3	3.8	53	1.3	1.0
Peas:						
no pod, 75g	●	8.5	3.5	62	5.1	1.1
boiled, 90g	●	9.0	4.0	71	6.0	1.4
canned, 90g	●	12.2	4.6	72	4.8	0.8
Peas, mushy, canned, 100g	●	13.8	1.8	81	5.8	0.7
Peas, processed, canned, 100g	●	17.5	4.8	99	6.9	0.7
See also: Petit pois						
See also under: Beans, Pulses						
and Cereals						
Peppers:						
green, raw, 40g	●	1.0	0.6	6	0.3	0.1
green, boiled, 50g	●	1.3	0.9	9	0.5	0.2
red, raw, 40g	●	2.6	0.6	13	0.4	0.2
red, boiled, 50g	●	3.5	0.9	17	0.6	0.2
yellow, raw, 40g	●	2.1	0.7	10	0.5	0.1
chilli, 15g	●	0.1	n/a	3	0.4	0.1

TIP: Roast a selection of Mediterranean vegetables in the oven.
Sprinkle a little balsamic salad dressing on top, scatter on some
pumpkin seeds and basil and crumble some feta cheese over the dish.

Food type	GI	Carb (g)	Fibre (g)	Cal (kcal)	Pro (g)	Fat (g)
Peppers, *contd*:						
jalapeños, 15g	●	0.5	–	3.3	0.2	0.04
Petit pois:						
fresh, 75g	●	13.1	3.1	75	5.2	0.6
frozen, boiled, 100g	●	5.5	4.5	49	5	0.9
Potatoes, Chips and Fries						
Chips, 150g:						
crinkle cut, frozen, fried	●	50.1	3.3	435	5.4	25
French fries, retail	●	51	3.2	420	4.9	23.2
homemade, fried	●	45.2	3.3	284	5.8	10
microwave chips	●	48.2	4.4	332	5.4	14.4
oven chips	●	44.7	3	243	4.8	6.3
straight cut, frozen, fried	●	54	3.6	410	6.2	20.2
Croquettes, fried in oil, 100g	●	21.6	1.3	214	3.7	13.1
Hash browns, 100g	●	24	–	190	3	9.8
Mashed potato, instant, 125g:						
made with semi-skimmed milk	●	18.5	1.2	88	3	1.5
made with skimmed milk	●	18.5	1.2	82	3	1.2
made with water	●	16.9	1.2	71	1.9	1.2
made up with whole milk	●	18.5	1.2	95	3	1.5
Potato fritters, 100g	●	17.2	1.3	174	2.2	10.7
Potato waffles, 100g	●	30.3	2.3	200	3.2	8.2

TIP: Potatoes shouldn't occupy more than a quarter of your plate.

Food type	GI	Carb (g)	Fibre (g)	Cal (kcal)	Pro (g)	Fat (g)
Potatoes, new, 100g:						
boiled, peeled	●	17.8	1.1	75	1.5	0.3
boiled in skins	●	15.4	1.5	66	1.4	0.3
canned	●	15.1	0.8	63	1.5	0.1
Potatoes, old, 90g:						
baked, flesh & skin	●	28.5	2.4	122	3.5	0.2
baked, flesh only	●	16.2	1.3	69	2.0	0.1
boiled, peeled	●	15.3	1.1	65	1.6	0.1
mashed with butter & milk	●	13.9	1.0	94	1.6	3.9
roast in oil/lard	●	23.3	1.6	134	2.6	4.0
Pumpkin, flesh only, boiled, 75g	●	1.6	0.8	10	0.4	0.2
Radicchio, 30g	●	0.5	0.5	4	0.4	0.1
Radish, red, 6	●	1.1	0.5	7	0.4	0.1
Radish, white/mooli, 20g	●	0.6	n/a	3	0.2	0.02
Ratatouille, canned, 115g	●	7.4	1.1	55	1.1	2.3
Salsify:						
flesh only, raw, 40g	●	4.1	1.3	11	0.5	0.1
flesh only, boiled, 50g	●	4.3	1.8	11	0.6	0.2
Shallots, 30g	●	1.0	0.6	6	0.4	0.2
Spinach:						
raw, one cup, 30g	●	0.5	0.6	7	0.8	0.2
boiled, 90g	●	0.7	1.9	17	2.0	0.7
frozen, boiled, 90g	●	0.4	1.9	19	2.8	0.7
Spring onions, bulbs & tops, 30g	●	0.9	0.4	7	0.6	0.2

Food type	GI	Carb (g)	Fibre (g)	Cal (kcal)	Pro (g)	Fat (g)
Sprouts: see Brussels Sprouts						
Squash:						
flesh only, 50g	●	1.1	0.2	6	0.2	0.1
flesh only, boiled, 75g	●	1.2	0.5	7	0.3	0.1
Swede, flesh only, boiled, 90g	●	2.0	0.6	10	0.3	0.1
Sweet potato, boiled, 90g	●	18.4	2.0	76	1.0	0.3
Sweetcorn, kernels, 80g:						
canned, drained, re-heated	●	21.3	1.1	97	2.3	1.0
canned, no salt, no sugar	●	13.4	2	62	2	–
Tomatoes:						
1 medium	●	4.7	1.1	26	1	0.4
canned, whole, 100g	●	3	0.7	16	1	0.1
cherry, 6	●	5.2	1.6	31	1.2	0.8
1 medium, fried in oil	●	7.8	1.4	137	1	10.3
sun-dried, 30g	●	3.3	1.9	63	1.3	4.9
paste, 2 tbsp	●	6	1	30	2	–
passata, 200g	●	9	0.4	50	2.8	0.2
chopped, canned, 200g	●	5	–	30	2.4	–
Turnip, flesh only, boiled, 60g	●	2.8	1.4	7	0.4	0.2
Water chestnuts, canned, 40g	●	3.0	n/a	12	0.4	–
Yam, flesh only, boiled, 90g	●	29.7	1.3	120	1.5	0.3
Zucchini: see Courgettes						

TIP: Buying organic makes a huge difference with vegetables. Not only are you avoiding pesticide residues, but they also tend to taste better.

VEGETARIAN

Only a few of the GI diet books specifically cater for vegetarians but the way of eating can easily be adapted to suit a vegetarian or vegan lifestyle, so long as the proportion of carbohydrate foods is kept low. The best substitute for meat, fish and eggs is soya protein or tofu. It easily takes on added flavours and can be made to resemble meat. Vegans may need to supplement their diet with vitamin B12.

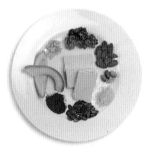

TIP: Many cardiologists recommend that we eat 25g of soya protein a day because of the benefits for our heart health. Even if you're not vegetarian, try using soya mince in your shepherds' pie or 'bolognese' sauce and, if you've never tried vegetarian burgers or sausages, you could be in for a treat.

Food type	GI	Carb (g)	Fibre (g)	Cal (kcal)	Pro (g)	Fat (g)
Baked beans with vegetable sausages, 200g	◐	24.2	5.8	204	11.2	7
Burgers:						
brown rice & tofu burgers, each	◐	10.1	3.2	184	12.2	10.6
carrot, peanut & onion burgers, each	◐	23.5	4.0	251	8.9	13.5
organic vegeburgers, each	◐	27.7	2.3	238	3.1	12.7
savoury burgers, each	◐	9.9	2.6	162	11.1	8.6
soya and black bean burgers, each	●	11.7	4.5	158	9.5	8.1
spicy bean burgers, each	●	23.2	3.5	241	5.9	13.9
vegetable burgers, each	◐	21	1.7	179	2.3	9.5
Cauliflower cheese, 100g	◐	22	–	365	18	23
Cheese, vegetarian:						
Double Gloucester, 25g		0.25	–	102	6.2	8.5
mild Cheddar, 25g		0.25	–	103	6.4	8.6
Red Leicester, 25g		0.25	–	100	8.1	8.4
Cornish pasty, each	●	37.3	2.0	452	11	28.9
Falafel, 4 (100g)	◐	23.3	7.6	220	8	10.5

TIP: Large Portobello mushrooms have the texture of tender meat and also a very low carb and GI count. Try making a mushroom 'steak' sandwich. Cook the mushrooms whole in garlic flavoured oil and choose a stoneground or Granary bread roll.

Food type	GI	Carb (g)	Fibre (g)	Cal (kcal)	Pro (g)	Fat (g)
Hummus, 2 tbsp	●	6.2	1.6	53	1.5	2.6
Lentils, 115g:						
green/brown, boiled	●	19.3	4.3	120	10	0.8
red, split, boiled	●	20	2.2	114	8.7	0.5
Macaroni cheese, individual	●	47	–	375	13	15
Nut roast, 100g:						
courgette & spiced tomato	●	12.5	4.9	208	11.7	12.3
leek, cheese & mushroom	●	13.2	4.1	240	13.2	14.9
Onions & garlic sauce, 100g	●	9.2	–	58	2.3	1.3
Pâté, 50g:						
chickpea & black olive	●	7.8	2.2	90	3.1	5.2
herb	●	3.0	–	83	3.5	8
herb & garlic	●	5.0	–	165	3.5	9
mushroom	●	3.5	–	100	3.5	8
red & green pepper	●	4.5	–	111	3	9
spinach, cheese & almond	●	3.2	1.2	86	3.6	6.6
Polenta, ready-made, 100g	●	15.7	–	71.9	1.6	0.3
Quorn, myco-protein, 100g	●	2	4.8	86	11.8	3.5
Ravioli in tomato sauce, (meatfree), 200g	●	28.8	1	150	4.8	1.6

TIP: Make kebabs by threading chunks of tofu, red and green peppers, courgette and mushroom onto a skewer. Coat in a mixture of tomato purée with paprika, cayenne pepper, garlic powder and black pepper then cook under a hot grill, turning frequently. Serve in pitta bread.

Food type	GI	Carb (g)	Fibre (g)	Cal (kcal)	Pro (g)	Fat (g)
Red kidney beans:						
small can (200g)	●	35.6	17	200	13.8	1.2
boiled, 115g	●	19.8	10.3	118	9.6	0.6
Rice drink, 240ml:						
calcium enriched	●	24	–	120	0.2	2.6
vanilla	●	24	–	118	0.2	2.4
Roast vegetable & tomato						
pasta, 97% fat-free, each	●	56	–	300	10	3.7
'Sausage' rolls, 100g	●	23.1	1.6	260	10.9	14.5
'Sausages', 100g (2 sausages)	●	8.6	1.2	252	23.2	13.8
spicy Moroccan	●	12.7	4.0	147	9.1	8.4
tomato & basil	●	9.3	3.2	147	8.6	9.8
Soya bean curd: *see* Tofu						
Soya chunks:						
flavoured, 100g	●	35	4	345	50	1
unflavoured, 100g	●	35	4	345	50	1
Soya curd: *see* Tofu						
Soya flour:						
full fat, 100g	●	23.5	11.2	447	36.8	23.5
low fat, 100g	●	28.2	13.5	352	45.3	7.2
Soya milk:						
banana flavour, 240ml	●	25.2	2.9	180	8.6	5

TIP: Vegetarian cheeses are not made with animal rennet, but they are still relatively high in fat so keep to small portions.

Food type	GI	Carb (g)	Fibre (g)	Cal (kcal)	Pro (g)	Fat (g)
Soya milk, *contd*:						
chocolate flavour, 240ml	●	23	3.6	173	8.6	5
strawberry flavour, 240ml	●	18.5	2.9	154	8.6	5
sweetened, 240ml	●	6	–	103	8.9	5
unsweetened, 240ml	●	1.2	0.5	62	5.8	3.8
Soya mince:						
flavoured, 100g	●	35	4	345	50	1
unflavoured, 100g	●	35	4	345	50	1
Spaghetti 'bolognese',						
(meatfree) 200g	●	26.2	1.4	172	6.2	4.8
Sweet pepper sauce, 100g	●	6	2.3	54	1.7	2.6
Tofu (soya bean curd), 100g:						
smoked	●	1.0	0.3	148	16	8.9
steamed	●	0.7	–	73	81	4.2
steamed, fried	●	2	–	261	23.5	17.7
tangy, marinated	●	2.0	0.4	70	7.9	3.4
Vegetable biryani, each	⬤	74	–	690	12	38
Vegetable granulated stock, 30g	●	11.9	0.3	60	2.5	0.3
Vegetable gravy granules, 50g	●	29.8	0.5	158	4.2	2.5
Vegetable sauce, 100ml	●	7	2.5	59	2	2.6
Vegetable stock cubes, each	●	4.6	0.2	28	1.2	0.5

TIP: Soya milk is lower in carbs than rice milk and therefore preferable on the GI diet, but choose brands that have added calcium to make sure you get enough of this important mineral.

Food type	GI	Carb (g)	Fibre (g)	Cal (kcal)	Pro (g)	Fat (g)
Vegetable pasty, each	●	29.9	1.8	188	4.4	5.7
Yoghurt-tofu organic, 100ml:						
peach & mango	●	20.5	1.5	128	4.8	2.8
red cherry	●	20.1	1.5	125	4.8	2.8
strawberry	●	19.5	0.3	135	4.8	0.3

TIP: Tofu is the best protein option for vegetarian GI dieters as it is low in carbs, low in saturated fats and cholesterol free, yet it contains a good range of B vitamins, calcium and iron.

FAST FOOD

Eating out at fast food restaurants is possible on a low GI diet but it will require a degree of self-control. Remove any crumbed or batter coatings on chicken or fish. Eat the burger without the bun. Don't order chips. Have a slice or two of pizza rather than the whole thing. Choose from the salad bar, if there is one, but avoid creamy mayonnaise sauces. Milkshakes and sweet fizzy drinks will send your blood sugar sky-high and the only low-GI drink will probably be still water.

TIP: The burger and chips meal shown above has 1066 calories, plus 57g of fat. The average woman who is *not* on a diet should eat around 1800 calories a day, while the average man should eat around 2200 calories and neither should eat more than 70g of fat. So after burger and chips they couldn't eat much else for the rest of the day.

Food type	GI	Carb (g)	Fibre (g)	Cal (kcal)	Pro (g)	Fat (g)
Burgers/Hotdogs						
BBQ pork in a bun	●	68.9	3.4	515	25.1	16.2
Bacon & egg in a bun	●	32.3	1.7	400	23.5	19.9
Bacon in a bun	●	32.3	1.7	290	15	11.2
Bacon cheeseburger	●	32.3	1.7	375	21.4	18.1
Cheeseburger, each	●	33.1	2.5	299	15.8	11.5
Frankfurter:						
in a bun	●	33.5	2.2	410	21.8	22.4
in a bun with cheese	●	33.5	2.2	455	21.8	25.9
Half-pounder	●	42.3	6.7	840	51.2	51.5
Hamburger (85g)	●	32.8	2.5	253	13.1	7.7
Quarter-pounder	●	37.1	3.7	423	25.7	19
with cheese	●	37.5	3.7	516	31.2	26.7
Spicy beanburger	●	68.7	15.9	535	16.1	22
Veggie burger	●	55.4	7.6	432	14.7	16.9
Chicken						
Chicken chunks & chips	●	68.3	4.2	645	21.4	31.6
Chicken dunkers	○	1.5	0.5	220	23.5	13.3
Chicken in a bun	●	42	1.9	435	16.3	22.2
Chicken nuggets (6)	○	11.5	2.1	253	18.6	14.8

TIP: Fast-food products will vary from outlet to outlet, but thin-crust pizzas will generally have a lower GI value than thicker crust ones, and you can reduce it further by eating a green salad on the side.

Food type	GI	Carb (g)	Fibre (g)	Cal (kcal)	Pro (g)	Fat (g)
Chicken strips, portion	◐	13.4	1	219	23.3	8
Chicken wings, portion	◐	3	2.3	466	40	32.7
Fish						
Cod, in batter, fried	●	11.7	0.5	247	16.1	15.4
Fish and chips	●	43.5	3.9	465	27.5	20.1
Fish in a bun	●	62.8	3.4	510	34.2	13.5
Plaice, in batter, fried	●	12	0.5	257	15.2	16.8
Rock salmon/dogfish, in batter, fried	●	10.3	0.4	295	14.7	21.9
Skate, in batter, fried	●	4.9	0.2	168	14.7	10.1
Pizza/Pasta						
Cannelloni, per portion	●	38.7	n/a	556	20.9	35.4
Deep-pan pizza, per slice:						
Margherita	●	31.5	n/a	256	13.5	8.5
Meat Feast	●	28	n/a	266	13	11.3
Supreme	●	29.6	n/a	257	13.1	9.6
Vegetarian	●	14.8	n/a	136	6.9	5.6
Lasagne, per portion	●	62.4	9.3	669	39.4	29.2
Medium-pan pizza, per slice:						
Ham & Mushroom	●	34	n/a	269	13	10.2

TIP: It would take a brisk 10km walk, 2½ hours playing tennis or 3 hours cycling to burn off all the calories in a quarter-pounder with cheese.

Food type	GI	Carb (g)	Fibre (g)	Cal (kcal)	Pro (g)	Fat (g)
Medium-pan pizza, contd:						
Ham & Pineapple	●	28	1.3	241	12.1	8.9
Margherita	●	37.5	n/a	291	14.4	10.2
Meat Feast	●	27.8	n/a	324	16.6	16.2
Supreme	●	26.5	n/a	297	13.7	14.6
Vegetarian	●	26.2	1.8	225	10.5	8.8
Thin crust, per slice:						
Cheese & Tomato	●	18.2	1.7	126	6.7	2.9
Full House	●	18.9	1.3	183	9.3	7.8
Mixed Grill	●	19.6	1.7	177	9	6.9
Pepperoni	●	20.6	1.4	187	9	7.6
Tandoori Hot	●	18.7	1.9	138	8.2	3.5
Thin crust, per pizza:						
American	●	87.3	n/a	753	35.3	32.4
Fiorentina	●	88.4	n/a	740	38.22	27.5
Four Cheese	●	87.2	n/a	636	29.4	22.1
Ham & Mushroom	●	87.4	n/a	665	34.9	22.8
Mushroom	●	87.5	n/a	627	30.1	20.6
Tomato Bake, per portion	●	92.9	5.5	653	27.1	21.6
Tortellini, per portion	●	91.9	n/a	1116	26.9	71.3
Side Orders						
Fries, regular portion	●	28.3	2.8	206	2.9	9
Fries, large portion	●	33.3	2.4	550	36.2	30.3
Garlic bread, portion	●	44.3	2.5	386	8	19.6

Food type	GI	Carb (g)	Fibre (g)	Cal (kcal)	Pro (g)	Fat (g)
Garlic bread with cheese, portion	●	49.5	3.3	618	25.6	35.3
Garlic mushrooms, portion	○	22.1	3.8	215	6.6	11.1
Hash browns	○	15.8	1.7	138	1.4	7.7
Potato skins, portion	●	51.4	4.7	570	7.6	37.1
Salade Niçoise, per portion	○	65	n/a	729	40	37
Drinks						
Milkshake, vanilla, regular, each	●	62.7	–	383	10.8	10.1
Dips						
BBQ Dip, portion	○	7.3	n/a	31	2.8	–
Cheesy Bites:						
Cheddar	○	28.7	n/a	319	8.5	18.9
Tomato & Cheddar	○	26.9	n/a	308	8.2	18.6
Garlic & Herb Dip, portion	○	6.21	n/a	280	1.29	27.75
Ranch Dip, portion	○	3.8	n/a	489	3.2	51
Meals						
All-day breakfast	●	46.2	3.8	710	31.4	44.3
Egg & chips	●	32.5	2.7	490	20.8	30.6

TIP: At the salad bar, choose green leafy vegetables and tomatoes. Avoid potato and sweetcorn salad and watch the dressings, which can bring the calorie and fat content of your salad to more than that of a burger meal.

Food type	GI	Carb (g)	Fibre (g)	Cal (kcal)	Pro (g)	Fat (g)
Mixed grill	●	46.4	3.9	770	36.7	49.1
Spicy Chicken Bake, portion	●	80.7	–	499	18.5	12.4
Sandwiches and Wraps						
Cheese & pickle, per pack	●	51	3.8	341	16	8.1
Cheese & tomato, per pack	●	43	3.6	306	21	5.5
Chicken & ham, per pack	●	34	3.2	294	25	6.4
Chicken salad wrap, per pack	●	46	3.2	307	18	5.7
Egg mayonnaise & cress, per pack	●	39	4.2	305	15	9.9
Egg salad, per pack	●	44	2	304	13	8.4
Flatbread:						
chicken tikka	●	24	1.4	172	11	3.6
Peking duck	●	29	1.9	169	7.4	2.6
spicy Mexican	●	23	3.7	156	7	4
tuna	●	19	1.3	123	8.8	1.3
Ham & Double Gloucester, per pack	●	35	4.5	307	20	9.7
Ham, cheese & pickle, per pack	●	33	5	296	22	8.4
Ham & cream cheese bagel, per pack	●	45	2.4	319	19	7
Mini sushi selection, per pack	●	53	4.1	293	9.6	4.7
Prawn mayonnaise, per pack	●	37	5.1	320	16	12
Roast chicken, per pack	●	31	2.4	288	24	7.5
Roast chicken salad, per pack	●	37	4.4	284	21	5.8

Food type	GI	Carb (g)	Fibre (g)	Cal (kcal)	Pro (g)	Fat (g)
Salmon & cucumber, per pack	●	39	3.5	327	18	11
Toasted tea cake & butter	●	35.3	1.2	250	5.8	9.9
Tuna & cucumber, per pack	●	43	3	323	20	7.9
Tuna & sweetcorn, per pack	●	48	3.4	317	19	5.4
Tuna melt, per pack	●	33	2.6	258	21	4.7

TIP: If you must have sandwiches, do everything you can to reduce the GI value. Choose wholemeal, rye or pumpernickel bread and a salad and lean protein filling with mayonnaise. There's advice on pages 232–5 about ways of making your own low-GI packed lunch.

Putting it into Practice

SOME GI COMPARISONS

Breads/crackers		Carbs with a meal	
Baguette	95	Easy-cook white rice	87
Gluten-free bread	90	Baked potatoes	85
Puffed rice cakes	77	Chips	75
Black rye bread	76	Risotto rice	69
Bagels	72	Taco shells	68
White bread	70	Polenta	68
Crumpet	69	Couscous	65
Croissant	67	Basmati rice	58
Cream crackers	65	Brown rice	55
Rye crispbread	63	Egg noodles	46
White rolls	61	Boiled potato	58
Granary bread	61	Durum wheat	
Stoneground bread	59	spaghetti	41
Pitta bread	57	Mung bean	
Sourdough bread	57	noodles	39
Oatcakes	54	Lentils	29
Rye bread	51	Chickpeas	28
Pumpernickel	50	Kidney beans	28
Fruit teabread	47	Pearl barley	25

Desserts

Rice pudding	81
Chocolate ice cream	68
Sponge cake with cream	67
Vanilla ice cream	61
Banana	52
Plain yoghurt	46
Orange	42
Custard	43
Low-fat fruit yoghurt	39
Peaches canned in juice	38
Fruit yoghurt	33
Strawberry mousse	32
Cherries	22

Drinks

Glucose drink	95
Beer	88
Lemon squash	66
Fizzy orange drink	68
Cola	53
Cranberry juice	52
Hot chocolate	51
Orange juice	50
Carrot juice	43
Apple juice	40
Tomato juice	38
Raspberry smoothie	33
Skimmed milk	32
Tea, black, unsweetened	0
Water	0

Fruits		Vegetables	
Watermelon	72	Parsnips	97
Pineapple	59	Broad beans	79
Banana	52	Beetroot	64
Mango	51	Sweetcorn	48
Grapes	46	Green peas	48
Orange	42	Carrots	47
Strawberries	40	Cabbage	0
Pear	38	Cauliflower	0
Apple	38	French beans	0
Prunes	29	Avocado	0
Grapefruit	25	Celery	0
Cherries	22	Lettuce	0

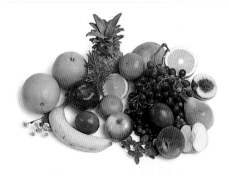

Breakfast foods		Snack foods	
Puffed wheat	80	Jelly beans	78
Cornflakes	77	Doughnut	76
White toast	70	Shortbread	64
Bran muffin	60	Muesli bar	61
Granary toast	61	Digestive biscuits	58
Swiss-style muesli	56	Blueberry muffin	59
Porridge	49	Oatcakes	57
Strawberry jam	51	Popcorn, plain	55
Orange juice	50	Plain crisps, salted	54
Full-fat cows' milk	27	Milk chocolate bar	49
Boiled egg	0	Corn chips, salted	42
Grilled bacon	0	Chocolate peanuts	33
		Cashews, salted	22

Note: GI values will vary between different manufacturers' brands. The scores given here are an average across a range of similar products.

MENU IDEAS FOR A LOW GI DIET

Most books on the GI diet give detailed menu plans and recipes. Below you will find ideas for some simple, easy-to-prepare meals. If creating your own meals, choose mainly items from the low- or no-GI items in the listings when you are trying to lose weight and introduce some yellow items when you reach your target weight.

Breakfast
- Plain yoghurt and an oat-based cereal bar
- Fresh fruit and nut platter – almonds are particularly good
- Porridge topped with dried blueberries or cherries
- Granary toast, unbuttered, with low-fat fromage frais and fruit conserve
- Grilled bacon and tomatoes
- One-egg omelette with mushrooms
- Bowl of unsweetened muesli and skimmed milk with dried apricots
- Rye crispbread with yeast extract and sliced tomato
- Banana and almond smoothie
- Buckwheat pancake with smoked salmon and lemon
- Cold lean ham and sliced pear
- Poached smoked haddock and egg with wholemeal toast

Lunch

- Wholemeal pasta with pesto and walnuts
- Salmon and mango salad with a soy sauce and sesame oil dressing
- Burritos with a bean and vegetable filling
- Two slices ciabatta with grilled Mediterranean vegetables and hummus

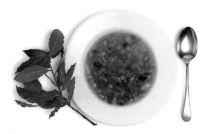

- Three bean soup with tomato base – French, kidney and haricot
- Falafels and salad
- Lentil, chicken and bacon salad
- Caesar salad with anchovies and poached egg but no croûtons
- Tomato, mozzarella and olive salad with a small wholemeal pitta
- Grilled herring with oatmeal coating and apple sauce

- Thai noodles with tofu, mangetouts and beansprouts
- Open pumpernickel sandwich with smoked salmon and cucumber

Snacks
- Crudités with hummus
- Two oatcakes
- Handful of almonds and raisins
- One medium fruit or small bunch grapes
- Two squares dark chocolate
- Small tub plain yogurt with fresh blueberries or raspberries
- One slice malt loaf, unbuttered
- Half an avocado with French dressing
- Small bowl cottage cheese with three chopped dried apricots
- Sixteen olives
- 2 plain digestives and a slice of low-fat cheese
- Mashed banana topped with sunflower seeds
- Cappuccino made with skimmed milk
- Fruit smoothie made with any fresh fruits that are in season, blended with ice

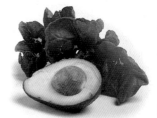

Dinner

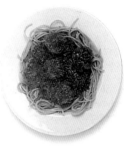

- Grilled pork and vegetable kebabs with 1tbsp basmati rice
- Sweet potato, cheese and leek mash with lean steak
- Spicy dahl with mushrooms and spinach
- Spaghetti with Bolognese sauce
- Peppers stuffed with couscous, sultanas and onions
- Fish cakes (more fish than potato) with fresh tomato sauce
- Baked potato topped with baked beans
- Pearl barley risotto with peas
- Chicken and bean enchiladas
- Grilled salmon fillet with chickpea and parsley purée
- Portobella mushrooms stuffed with wholemeal crumbs, herbs and lean bacon
- Chilli con carne
- Fresh tuna steak served with a mixed salad, green beans, anchovies and chopped hard-boiled egg
- Chicken or vegetable curry with basmati rice

Desserts

- Pears cooked in red wine and cinnamon
- Stewed rhubarb with blueberries
- Gooseberry and ginger crumble with oats
- Banana fool made with Greek-style yoghurt
- Halved peaches with toasted flaked almonds
- Stewed dried apricots, cherries and cranberries
- Vanilla ice cream with sieved strawberries
- Summer pudding
- Lemon jelly with sliced oranges
- Baked apple filled with sultanas and cinnamon
- Baked egg custard
- Pineapple slice with passion fruit topping

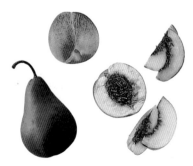

EATING OUT

Once you understand the basic principles of a GI diet, you should be able to look through the menu and find low-GI dishes in virtually any kind of restaurant. It's certainly easier than if you were following a calorie-counting, carb-counting or low-fat regime. You may have to ask the waiter some pertinent questions about ingredients and how sauces were made, and you might decide to change the accompanying chips for a green salad or extra vegetables, but most restaurants should be able to accommodate you.

The cuisines are listed in alphabetical order by their country of origin, starting with traditional British fare. The last section is on packed meals. Many people take packed lunches to work as it is usually more economical and, for those a GI diet, it is the best way to ensure you are sticking by the rules while getting some variety in your diet at the same time. For advice on eating in fast-food restaurants, see pages 200-6.

British

Select good-quality basic foods that have been simply cooked and you won't go far wrong. Follow Azmina Govindji's suggestion and, as you visualise the plate, say to yourself 'VVPC' (Veggie, veggie, protein, carbs). You might decide to order an extra veg and forego the potatoes – and remember that you'll fall off the wagon if you venture into the territory of pies, pastries and puds.

Low GI choices
- Porridge and oatcakes
- Wholemeal toast
- Grilled fish, preferably oily fish like salmon, herrings or kippers
- Poached smoked haddock with poached egg
- Dover sole
- Grilled lean meat (cut off any visible fat)
- Simple roasts like beef, game, pork – but no crackling
- Grilled liver and bacon

High GI choices to avoid
- Full English breakfast with fried bread
- Side orders of bread or rolls
- Pastry or potato-topped pies, such as steak & kidney, shepherd's, fish
- Battered or crumbed fish

- Yorkshire pudding
- Chips and anything fried
- Haggis, neeps and mashed potato
- Traditional puddings like steamed syrup sponge or spotted dick and custard
- Beer

Chinese

This is not the easiest cuisine to choose from when following a GI diet. Rice is a Chinese staple and it is nearly always the short-grain, sticky kind which has the highest GI. Noodles aren't any better, apart from the cellophane kind which can be hard to come by. Small quantities of monosodium glutamate (MSG) are often added to Chinese food to enhance flavours; note that this is a high-carb and high-GI ingredient. Try to choose a restaurant which states it does not use MSG.

Low GI choices

- Clear soups
- Stir-fried vegetables, like beansprouts, mangetouts and cabbage
- Baked and grilled fish
- Stir fried chicken or beef but no thickened sauces
- Boiled cellophane noodles (made from mung beans) – but not crispy ones, which have been fried

- Dishes made with tofu (bean curd)
- Savoury sauces such as soy, oyster sauce, ginger and garlic
- Jasmine tea

High GI choices to avoid
- Any white rice
- Any noodles apart from cellophane
- Sesame prawn toasts
- Dumplings (dim sum)
- Spring rolls
- Sweet and sour dishes
- Crispy or Peking duck with pancakes
- Toffee apples or bananas

French
It seems odd that a nation whose cuisine is reputedly based on cream and butter and consumption of daily baguettes and croissants should not have the same level of obesity as the British. The answer may lie in the omnipresent French street markets. There is hardly a village that does not have at least a weekly market with its stalls piled high with seasonal fruits and vegetables, and these form the base of much French cooking. When eating in a French restaurant, the main things to avoid on a GI diet are cream sauces, pastry and tarts.

Low GI choices

- French onion soup – ask for it without the croûte (toasted bread slice) and cheese
- Salads with oily fish, such as Niçoise
- Cassoulet – a casserole with meat and beans
- Grilled entrecôte or tournedos steak 'au poivre' (with ground black pepper)
- Moules marinières (mussels in a wine and onion sauce)
- Crudités (raw vegetable strips)
- *Truite aux amandes* (grilled trout with almonds)

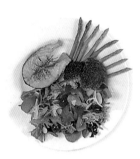

High GI choices to avoid

- Creamy soups and sauces
- Anything *en croûte* (baked in pastry)
- *Pommes* and *pommes frîtes* (potatoes and chips)
- Tarts and quiches
- Crêpes
- Profiteroles
- Sorbets and ice creams

Greek

It would be possible to eat a whole meal based on mezze – the little appetiser dishes – but some of the meat stews and kebabs are low GI too. If you are by the coast, eat the local fish, grilled. The Greeks use monounsaturated olive oil to cook in and fresh lemons squeezed on top for extra flavour.

Low GI choices

- Greek salad with tomato, cucumber and feta cheese and a small wholewheat pitta bread
- Hummus, taramasalata and tzatziki with raw vegetable dippers
- *Gigantes* – large butter beans usually in a tomato sauce
- *Fasioli plaki* – a bean casserole
- Souvlaki – meat and vegetable skewers/kebabs.
- Grilled fish and seafood with lemon
- Kleftiko and Stifado – meat casseroles

High GI choices to avoid

- Dolmades – rice stuffed vine leaves
- Moussaka, which is made with potato and a creamy topping

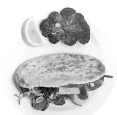

- Spanakopitta – spinach and feta wrapped in filo pastry
- Calamari – squid rings or baby squid deep fried in batter
- Meatballs and sausages
- Baklava – pastries made with honey.

Indian

Most Indian restaurants have a good selection of vegetable dishes, which are usually low GI. Tandoori dishes are dry fried and are served with salads, so make a good GI meal. Lentil and chickpea dishes are fine but the rice and breads that normally accompany curries are not. Yoghurt is usually full-fat so should be eaten in moderation.

Low GI choices

- Tandoori and Balti dishes with salad or basmati rice
- Baked or grilled meat dishes, rather than deep-fried
- Vegetable dishes – *bhindi bhaji* (ladies' fingers or okra), *sag* (spinach), *gobi* (cauliflower), *brinjal* (aubergine)
- Raita (cucumber and yoghurt), tomato and coriander chutney, chilli and lime pickle
- *Dahl* (lentil dishes)
- *Chana* (chickpea dishes)
- Fresh guava

High GI choices to avoid

- Breads – naan, chapattis, puri, paratha, roti, poppadums
- Deep-fried appetisers with batter or pastry – pakora, samosas
- Rice dishes – birianis, pilaus and rice as an accompaniment.
- Dishes containing potato (*aloo*)
- Dishes containing coconut
- All Indian desserts and ice creams – *kulfi, gulab jamun*

Italian

This is one of the easiest cuisines for a low GI diet. There are usually plenty of antipasti and salad dishes to choose from as well as grilled fish and meats. A slice of thin-based pizza or a small portion of spaghetti with lots of vegetable sauce can be chosen occasionally but don't eat a whole plateful – pasta should only fill a side plate, or a quarter of a dinner plate. Choose the fresh fruit option for dessert.

Low GI choices

- Thin soups (*brodo*)
- Antipasti – grilled vegetables, lean cold meats, Parma ham and melon, olives, artichokes, mushrooms
- Salads – rocket, fennel, green beans, tricolore (avocado, mozzarella and tomato)

- Grilled fish, chicken or veal
- I slice of thin-based pizza with vegetable, tomato and onion topping
- Small portion pasta (must be durum wheat, not egg pasta) with vegetable sauce and no grated cheese
- Fresh fruit in season

High GI choices to avoid
- Garlic bread and breadsticks
- Egg pasta with creamy and cheese sauces
- Risottos
- Polenta (made with maize flour)
- Deep-pan or medium-pan pizzas
- Meat cooked in breadcrumbs – *scaloppini*
- Desserts like *gelato* (ice cream), *tiramisu, panna cotta*

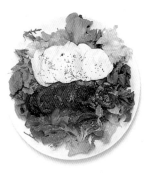

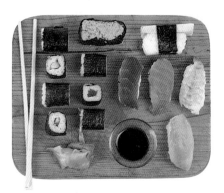

Japanese

Trays of sushi are now a familiar sight in our super-markets as well as in Japanese restaurants. Although they are fish-based, they also contain a high proportion of rice, which makes them unsuitable for a low GI diet. Sashimi, however, is a great choice, full of protein and healthy fatty acids. Generally try to avoid rice and noodles, apart from cellophane noodles, and choose green vegetables like spinach or beans, or shiitake mushrooms. Teppenyaki restaurants are a good choice as the menu consists of plainly grilled fish or meat and you can see the food cooked in front of you.

Low GI choices

- Sashimi – raw, fresh fish pieces served with wasabi (hot horseradish)
- Tofu dishes
- Mixed fish casseroles
- Steamed fish or chicken
- *Sukiyaki* – meat and vegetables with tofu
- *Shabu-shabu* – meat and vegetables cooked (by you) in a stock pot on your table
- Soy bean casserole

High GI choices to avoid

- Sushi
- Vegetable tempura (deep-fried in batter)
- Anything with rice or potatoes
- Anything coated in breadcrumbs and fried
- Anything in rice wrappers
- Anything with *miso* (fermented beans) or *mirin* (sweetened saké).

Mexican

Beans (*frijoles*) are low-GI options used in soups and meat dishes in Mexican cooking, but avoid refried beans (*frijoles refritos*), which have been cooked in oil. Tomato salsa and guacamole are tasty side orders, to eat with meat or fish dishes. Unfortunately, the staple Mexican main courses with meat and cheese rolled inside tortillas are all off the GI scoreboard, and it's not so satisfying to eat chilli without the rice.

Low GI choices

- Guacamole dip with vegetables
- *Ceviche* – raw fish salad with avocado
- *Sopa de frijol Negro* – black bean soup
- *Salpicon* (shredded cold beef salad)
- Chilli con carne, but no rice.
- Grilled fish, chicken or meat.
- Salsas

High GI choices to avoid

- Any dish made with tortillas – quesadillas, enchiladas, tacos, burritos, chimichangas, fajitas
- Nachos (corn chips)
- *Torta* – Mexican filled rolls or sandwiches.
- Rice (*arroz*) dishes
- *Mole* – thick rich sauces often darkened with chocolate
- *Postres* (pastries and desserts)

Middle Eastern

This is another cuisine where a meal can be made from mezze – the range of appetiser dishes. Low GI beans, nuts and lentils are frequently used as an ingredient. Side salads are always available and they should have a range of grilled meats and fish.

Low GI choices

- *Baba Ghanoush* – grilled and pureed aubergine with tahini (sesame seed paste) and lemon
- *Fool Akhdar* – fresh broad bean salad with coriander
- *Falafel* – rissoles made with chickpeas
- Hummus
- Kebabs, such as *Sheesh Tawoo* – chicken kebabs – but served without bread or rice
- *Kefta meshwi* – meatballs cooked on skewers

High GI choices to avoid

- Couscous
- Tabbouleh – cracked wheat salad
- Vine leaves stuffed with rice
- Potato dishes, such as *Batata Hara*
- *Fatayer* – savoury pastries made with cheese, spinach and pine kernels
- *Baklava* – honey pastries – and all cakes

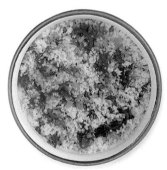

Spanish

A tapas bar is a good place to eat on a GI diet. Dishes are sometimes laid out along the bar, so you can see the ingredients at a glance, and portions are small, saucer sizes. However, paella, the classic rice-based Spanish dish, is sadly off-limits.

Low GI choices
- Anchovies in vinegar
- Olives and nuts
- Grilled meats and salads
- Pickled chillies
- Gazpacho – chilled tomato and pepper soup – but with no croutons
- *Pollo en Pepitoria* – chicken braised with almonds
- Grilled fish and seafood

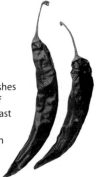

High GI choices to avoid
- Paella
- Any rice- or potato-based dishes
- *Churros* – deep-fried strips of sweet batter, eaten at breakfast time
- Spanish omelette (made with potatoes)
- Flan (caramel custard)

Thai

Rice and noodles are served with everything. Try to keep to the cellophane noodles made from mung beans. Salads can be delicious mixtures of tropical fruits with fish and meat. Satays of chicken and meat are always available, but keep the portion of peanut sauce small.

Low GI choices

· Prawn and papaya salad
· Mango and salmon salad
· Clear soups with vegetables and chicken or fish – the classic is *tom yam pla* with fish and straw mushrooms
· Satay with peanut sauce
· Steamed mussels with basil
· Green and red curries but no rice
· Beef or chicken salads
· Steamed tofu dishes
· Tropical fruits

High GI choices to avoid

· Soups with rice or noodles, like *pho*
· Fried or crispy noodles (*sen* means noodles)
· Rice based dishes (*khao* means rice, and *khao man* is coconut rice)
· Spring rolls

Packed Lunches

If packed meals are a regular part of your lifestyle, it would be a good idea to invest in some quality packaging: different sizes of lidded plastic boxes and beakers, a thermos jug or two and a small insulated bag which will keep foods hot as well as chilled, depending on the weather. Disposable plates, cutlery, wet cloths and paper napkins will make the meal more civilised.

To some people, packed lunches are synonymous with sandwiches, but going heavy on bread is not a good idea on a GI diet so restrict them to only once a week. Make sure the bread is high in fibre and the fillings are ultra-healthy. Choose open sandwiches to reduce the bread content. Salads travel well in plastic boxes if the dressing is carried separately, and most fruits will survive the few hours until they are eaten.

Low- to medium-GI breads that travel well

- Wholegrain or granary, sliced
- Wholemeal pitta
- Tortilla wraps
- Linseed rye bread
- Oatcakes
- Rye crispbreads
- Pumpernickel

Low-GI sandwich fillings

- Prepared salad vegetables: baby spinach, sliced tomatoes or halved baby tomatoes, sliced cucumber, grated carrot, shredded crisp lettuce, rocket, celery, courgette
- Low-fat cottage cheese
- Lean cooked skinless chicken
- Canned oily fish: tuna, sardines, salmon
- Smoked mackerel pâté
- Lean roast beef or ham
- Taramasalata
- Nut butter: almond, peanut or hazelnut

Low-GI salads

- Grilled Mediterranean vegetables with olive oil and balsamic vinegar
- Beansprouts, canned chickpeas, spring onion and watercress with a ginger and soy dressing

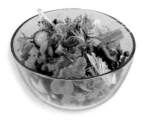

- Raw vegetable crudités – carrots, celery, cauliflower and broccoli florets, peppers, radishes – with a dip such as hummus or tzatziki
- Broad beans and peas with lean ham
- Cooked pearl barley mixed with radishes, spring onions, avocado, pumpkin seeds, chopped dried fruit and crumbled feta cheese

- Niçoise, with tuna and hard-boiled egg
- Mixed beans – French, red kidney and borlotti – with canned tuna and thin red onion rings, in a vinaigrette dressing
- Goat's cheese on rocket, with cherry tomatoes, red peppers, basil and pine nuts

Low- or medium-GI snacks

Olives, dried fruit, whole shelled unsalted nuts (almonds, walnuts or pecans), home-made cereal bars or oaten biscuits.

Fruits in season
- Fresh cherries are the lowest GI fruit
- Fresh raspberries come a close second, as do any berry fruits which do not need sweetening
- Figs are easy to eat if you pack a knife
- Fresh sliced peaches or apricots

- Red or green
  grapes
- Apples and
  pears in
  season
- Citrus fruits

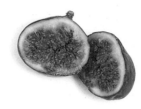

Low-GI drinks

- Bottled water is the easiest and best
  drink to pack
- Hot beef or yeast extract in a flask
- A simple chilled soup for summer can be made by
  mixing tomato juice with plain yoghurt, seasoning
  well and keeping in the flask with one or two ice
  cubes
- Fruit smoothies made with berry fruits

High-GI foods to avoid

- Any confectionery
- Bags of crisps and savoury snacks, no matter how
  small
- Salted nuts
- Sweet fizzy drinks
- Sweet biscuits and cakes
- Most sandwiches
- Chips or fried foods

FURTHER READING

General Nutrition

Bodyfoods for Busy People, Jane Clarke, 2004

Collins Gem Calorie Counter, 2004

Collins Gem What Diet?, 2005

Collins Gem Healthy Eating, 1999

Collins Gem Carb Counter, 2004

Eat Well, Live Well series, recipe books, various authors

Fat is a Feminist Issue, Susie Orbach, 1998

Food Pharmacy, Jean Carper, 2000

A Good Life, Leo Hickman, 2005

Greek Doctor's Diet, Fedon Alexander Lindberg, 2005

Jane Clarke's Bodyfoods Cookbook: Recipes for Life, Jane Clarke, 2001

L is for Label: How to Read Between the Lines on Food Packaging, Amanda Ursell, 2004

Nutrition for Life, Ian W. Campbell, 2005

Patrick Holford's New Optimum Nutrition Bible, Patrick Holford, 2004

Think Well to be Well, Azmina Govindji, 2002

The Vegetarian Low-Carb Diet, Rose Elliott, 2005

Vitamins and Minerals Handbook, Amanda Ursell et al, 2001

You Are What You Eat Cookbook, Dr Gillian McKeith, 2005

The GI Diet

The GI Diet, by Rick Gallop, 2004

The GI Diet – Shopping and Eating Out Pocket Guide, by Rick Gallop, 2005

Living the GI Diet: To Maintain Healthy, Permanent Weight Loss, Rick Gallop, 2004

The GI Guide, Rick Gallop and Hamish Renton, 2005

The Low GI Diet, by Jennie Brand-Miller & Kaye Foster-Powell with Joanna McMillan-Price, 2004

The Complete Guide to GI Values, Jennie Brand-Miller, Kaye Foster-Powell & Dr Susanna Holt, 2004

The Low GI Life Plan, by Jennie Brand-Miller & Kaye Foster-Powell, 2004

The Low GI Diet, Jennie Brand-Miller, 2005

The High-Energy Cookbook, by Rachael Anne Hill, 2004

Easy GI Diet, by Helen Foster, 2004

The GI Plan, by Azmina Govindji & Nina Puddefoot, 2004

The G-Index Diet, by Richard Podell & William Proctor, 1994

Antony Worrall Thompson's GI Diet, by Antony Worrall Thompson, 2005

The Fat Busting GI Angel, Gunter Schaule, 2003

The Simple 0–10 GI Diet, Azmina Govindji and Nina Puddefoot, 2005

The Healthy Low GI and Low Carb Diet, Charles Clark, Maureen Clark, 2005

USEFUL WEBSITES

www.bodyfoods.com
www.weightlossresources.co.uk/diet/gi_diet
www.glycaemicindex.com (Jennie Brand-Miller's Australian website)
www.gisymbol.com.au (another Australian website)
www.diabetes.org.uk/faq/gi
www.waitrose.com/food_drink/nutrition/healthy eating/glycaemicindex.asp
www.gidiet.com (Rick Gallop's website)
www.ivillage.co.uk (the Tesco website for diet queries)
www.healthnet.org.uk (Coronary Prevention Group)
www.sainsburys.com/healthyeating
www.asda.com
www.edietsuk.co.uk (also used by Tesco)

USEFUL ADDRESSES

British Dietetic Association
5th Floor, Charles House
148/9 Great Charles Street
Queensway
Birmingham B3 3HT
www.bda.uk.com

British Heart Foundation
14 Fitzhardinge Street
London W1H 6DH
020 7935 0185

British Nutrition Foundation
High Holborn House
52-54 High Holborn
London WC1V 6RQ
020 7404 6504

Diabetes UK
10 Parkway
London NW1 7AA
Careline 0845 1202960
Or 020 7424 1000 and ask to
be transferred to the Careline

Coronary Prevention Group
020 7927 2125
www.healthnet.org

Institute for Optimum Nutrition
Blades Court, Deodar Road
London SW15 2NU
020 88779993
No nutrition advice given but they will
recommend a nutritionist

Women's Health Concern
PO Box 2126
Marlow
Bucks SL7 2PU
Tel. 0845 1232319 to speak to a nurse
or 01628 488065 for other information
www.womens-health-concern.org